Exercise with Type 1 Diabetes

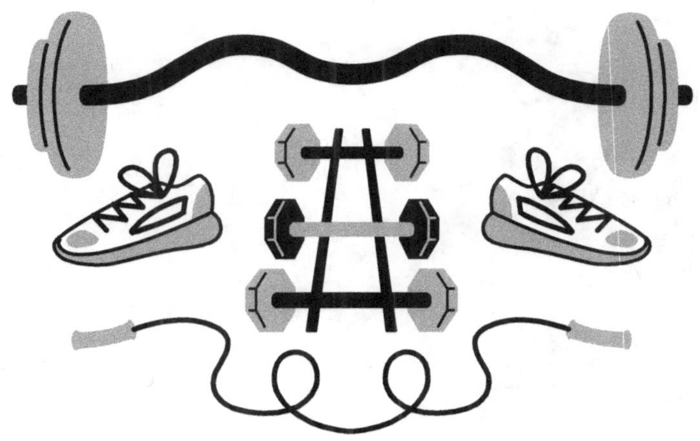

by Ginger Vieira

Foreword by Sheri R. Colberg, Ph.D.

Published by Ginger Vieira

GingerVieira.com

©2023, Ginger Vieira

All Rights Reserved

Cover and interior design by Brent Burdick

townbench.com

ISBN: 9798386208493

For more information, visit GingerVieira.com

Dedication and gratitude

I dedicate this book to my incredibly supportive husband, Karl Richardson. He listens to me wax poetically about type 1 diabetes nearly every day during our dog walks. He reviews insulin adjustments I've made — and how it all worked out. He discusses insulin adjustments I haven't made yet, but I might — and why. He has frequently stopped me from taking a potentially aggressive bolus with a gentle reminder like, "Umm, I think you should take a smaller dose." I am so grateful for his handsome daily support.

I must express a big thank you to Manny Hernandez — a person living with T1D who has dedicated decades of his life to advocating for people with all types of diabetes. In the midst of a conversation on social media with someone else, I mentioned that I wanted to write this book. Suddenly, Manny joined the conversation and basically suggested I set a deadline. So I did. And I wouldn't dare disappoint Manny Hernandez.

Thank you to Samantha, Pete, Alyssa, Karl, and Sheri for your thoughtful editing!

And lastly, **thank you to the talented Brent Burdick** for making this book a beautiful pile of pages we can hold in our hands.

Self-publishing takes a village!

Contents

Foreword

If you're looking for an informative and easy-to-follow read about how to be physically active with type 1 diabetes, look no further than this latest book by prolific author and journalist, Ginger Vieira. Need to know the impact of doing CrossFit training in the early morning? The answer is here. Need to know what happens when you exercise right after a meal? Again, you'll learn what you need to know from Ginger to handle it like a champ.

One of the biggest challenges that everyone who takes insulin faces is how to be active and keep blood glucose (sugar) in balance. If you have too much insulin in your blood, it may go too low. If you don't have enough, you can end up too high. It can be frustrating when you are unable to keep it balanced and exhilarating when you do. But all of us can use some help from someone else who has been there — to cut down on our trial-and-error period and reduce our learning curve, if nothing else. That's why you need to read this book.

Even at a relatively young age (especially compared to me), Ginger has done all types of athletic training. She has participated in competitive weight training and everyday aerobic activities that include chasing young kids. Her personal examples sprinkled throughout the book are ones that the majority of people with type 1 diabetes can relate to and learn from, and she backs up her experiences with an admirable understanding of how the body works with exercise when you have type 1 diabetes. She is a treasure trove of useful information, and you need to stop everything you are doing right now and read this book! You won't be sorry.

Sheri R. Colberg, Ph.D. Diabetes Motion Expert
Professor Emerita (Exercise Science), Old Dominion University
Person living (and exercising) with type 1 diabetes since 1968

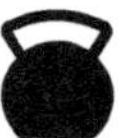

Exercise didn't come easily to me

It's easy to make a lot of assumptions when you see a visually "fit" person. It's also easy to assume they just have a skinny body type, that it's easy for them to maintain, that they've always been fit, that they've never been overweight, and that they couldn't possibly have the challenges you have.

I used to make these assumptions. After struggling with my weight between the ages of 15 to 28 years old, I realized that a lot of it actually comes down to a variety of daily choices and habits.

My T1D diagnosis story — in a nutshell

I was diagnosed with type 1 diabetes in 1999 at 13 years old after reading most of my symptoms on the posterboard of my classmate who had chosen "diabetes" as the topic for our 7th-grade health fair. I told my parents I thought I had diabetes. They said, "No, no, no. Only old people get that."

A week later, I burst into tears because I felt so lousy — losing weight, blurry vision, desperately thirsty, peeing constantly, and wondering why my legs felt so heavy and tired. They took me to my pediatrician and my diagnosis was obvious with a blood sugar over 500 mg/dL.

Within the first day or so of my hospitalization, I had begun to feel *really* sorry for myself. Crying, crying, crying. But I had an epiphany, truly, amidst my tears. I suddenly realized that *no one* has an easy life. No one.

I started thinking of my friends and the tremendous challenges and suffering they'd faced by the mere age of 13. Cancer, leukemia, sexual assault, hemophilia, depression, losing a parent to cancer, losing a parent to mental illness, losing part of their brain to a tumor. I just realized: life is challenging for everyone and type 1 diabetes is now one of my challenges.

I left the hospital with insulin and the determination to simply do the best I could.

Neglecting myself caught up with me

I was not a particularly athletic child. I tried team sports but was never very good at any of them.

As a teenager, I jogged regularly, walked in the woods a lot with my dog, and often walked a couple of miles to my job. Instead of school sports, I worked nearly 30 hours a week with my friends at the local movie theater.

By the time I graduated high school, I was about 20 pounds overweight. By the time I finished my freshman year of college, I was easily 30 pounds overweight. I simply wasn't taking care of myself. I wasn't connected to my body. I wasn't thinking about my nutrition. My A1c was usually somewhere between 6.7 to 7.3 percent — and considering CGMs didn't really exist yet, I considered that more than good enough. My healthcare team was thrilled with my A1c and they never commented on my weight.

It wasn't until the end of my junior year in college when my A1c spiked over 8 percent that I was startled into noticing my lack of wellness. I was thriving academically, loving my pursuit of a professional writing degree, serving as Editor-in-Chief of the college newspaper, acting in the Improv Comedy Troupe, and spending time with great friends — but I was truly neglecting every other part of my physical wellness.

I was at least 30 pounds overweight. I was eating gluten regularly (oh, I have celiac disease, by the way). I was stress-eating Chinese food or chocolate-glazed doughnuts whenever I felt overwhelmed or upset. (I was probably stress-eating other things but those two items really stand out in my memory!) I was still doing my best to manage my blood sugar but my best couldn't keep up with my not-so-helpful habits.

But that spike in my A1c got my attention. It scared me. I'd never seen it that high before and I knew there was only one obvious explanation: I really hadn't been taking care of myself.

Discovering my love of exercise

The summer between my junior and senior years, I got down to business.

While working as an assistant manager at the movie theater back in my hometown, I started going to power yoga classes several times a week because my grandfather's wife's daughter had her own studio. And I joined a gym and started teaching myself basic weightlifting. Using what I'd learned from my brothers and an old Schwarzenegger book of my father's, I was lifting weights every other day. I also started walking almost daily. And I dramatically changed my diet.

My diet wasn't anything crazy — this was long before the ketogenic/low-carb craze had begun. It was simply more real food and less junk. I remember eating oatmeal for breakfast, yogurt and nuts for lunch, and big bowls of microwaved veggies.

I didn't stop stress eating immediately, but I started being more aware of when and why I was doing it. I started asking myself, "Is this actually helping me feel less stressed? Less overwhelmed?" (The answer was a big no.)

By the end of that summer, I returned to Burlington, VT for my senior year of college feeling *in charge* of my life. My A1c came down into the high 6s. I had lost 15 pounds and gained noticeable muscle in my arms. One of my friends looked at me and said, *"Who are you?"* after asking me to flex my new muscles. The change in my self-esteem was impossible to miss.

I felt capable. I realized my body could be strong. I realized my body could feel powerful. It was the first time I felt truly connected to my body.

I joined a gym near my college town and hired a personal trainer to help me take my weightlifting knowledge to the next level. I was using all of my free time to learn *more* about lifting weights and Ashtanga power yoga. I also started walking every day at 6 a.m. with my new friends from the gym before college classes at 9 a.m.

By the end of my senior year, I had become a certified Ashtanga yoga instructor and certified personal trainer. During the next year, I was teaching my own yoga classes daily and training dozens of clients in the gym. I was also training intensely with my powerlifting coach. Between 2009 and 2011, I had over a dozen records in drug-free amateur power-lifting. At a competing bodyweight of 148 pounds, my best lifts included a 315-pound deadlift, a 190-pound bench press, and a 265-pound squat.

I felt very powerful and very proud of what my body could do.

I had discovered that I was athletic after all. It wasn't just my brothers! It was me, too. I had the potential to kick some butt with my own muscles and bones.

How was I managing my blood sugar? My daily insulin needs had gradu-ally dropped from 32 units of Lantus to 18 units. Since I wasn't wearing a CGM — which means I was likely pricking my finger 4 to 5 times per day — my overall target range was inevitably much broader than target ranges today.

Based on my A1c, my average blood sugar was around 158 mg/dL. My ap-proach to preventing lows wasn't much more than eating 15 to 30 grams of carbs before exercising. I don't recall devastating lows or confusing highs, but I was likely between 150 to 200 mg/dL on a regular basis which certainly helps avoid big swings during exercise.

Fibromyalgia fun!

Amidst the super intense Russian deadlifting programs, I believe the stress of my powerlifting training triggered what was eventually diag-nosed as fibromyalgia. What the heck is fibromyalgia? Honestly, they still don't know. It might be an autoimmune condition but there are many theories. For me, it is a combination of intense pain and intense exhaustion — triggered by any fun intense activity.

Within just a few years of my powerlifting pursuits, I had to abruptly stop because the pain throughout most of my joints, my lower back, my hips, my wrists, and my neck was too intense to bear.

Fortunately, my relationship with food was in a very peaceful place. I lost about 25 pounds of powerlifting-related muscle and chub while I tried to figure out what was causing so much pain. I was happy to let go of the bulky weight I carried from powerlifting.

By the time I got a proper diagnosis, the muscles in my neck were spasming so intensely that I could barely turn my head. The muscles in my hands could barely grip the knob of my front door. I couldn't lift a pot off the stove. I couldn't type for more than a few minutes before my hands started cramping with pain.

For several months, I was quite afraid. Afraid I couldn't work. Afraid I couldn't function.

I was able to rule out all the obvious issues (Lyme's, rheumatoid arthritis, multiple sclerosis, etc.) with simple blood tests but I was still being generally dismissed by doctors. On paper, I looked pretty darn healthy. Fortunately, I knew in my gut that something was truly wrong.

I fired the lousy and lazy doctors and finally found a great one.

This rheumatologist was the first to look at all of my symptoms together and *believe me*. She said, "I think you have fibromyalgia and I'm going to prescribe you cyclobenzaprine. Also, you need to start exercising like a grandmother — nothing intense."

That last bit was pretty heartbreaking for someone with a passion for intense weightlifting!

Cyclobenzaprine is a muscle relaxant — and it gave me my life back! Long story short: I spent the next two years letting my body calm down with support from cyclobenzaprine. The next two years after that, I started experimenting with different types of exercise. I quickly learned that any exercise that produces a lot of lactic acid (like intense weightlifting or hiking — that burning sensation in your muscles when they are working hard) triggers my extreme fibro-exhaustion. (I don't know why. I just know it's true for me!)

I was truly afraid to exercise for quite a while because of the pain and the debilitating exhaustion that would follow. I had to really reset my idea of what exercise looked like. I couldn't do *anything* intensely or for very long without a flare-up.

I could've given up. Instead, I was determined to figure out what I could still do. I had no particular goals beyond "just be active" and "don't trigger flare-ups."

In that process, I was actually gradually increasing what my body could still do!

Gradually, I realized I was actually rebuilding my body's tolerance for exercise. I can do things today that would have left me dysfunctional for days. Patience. Persistence. Patience.

Adapt. Improvise. Overcome.

In fact, my father had a little mantra that suits this situation quite perfectly. He would often tell me: "Adapt, Improvise, and Overcome!"

"Gin, you've gotta A-I-O!" he'd say with the energy of a man who bicycled 70 miles most days at 5 a.m.

It's been eight years since I was diagnosed with fibromyalgia and I'm proud to share that I truly feel athletic again. I can jump rope for 40 minutes. I can lift light-to-medium weights. I can go on long daily walks with my fella. I skate, sled, and play with my kids.

I can run 5K events, and jog a few miles on a nearly daily basis. I have my yellow belt in karate and can spar intensely with my classmates of higher belts. It's *fun*. It's the perfect combination of the intensity I love without much lactic acid. In a couple of months, I'll be competing in my first karate tournament! (And yet, a yoga class is very painful and I avoid it like the plague.)

But it took time and patience to get here. Leaving my pride and my ego at the door.

Staying active still requires daily careful thought. Every now and then, I accidentally overdo it and trigger exhaustion flare-ups, requiring me to take long naps in the middle of the day. The only cure for the exhaustion is sleep. Sometimes it takes a day to recover. Sometimes it takes a few days.

I've weaned myself completely off cyclobenzaprine. I manage my joint pain by avoiding certain activities and wearing a compression wrap on my wrists for large parts of the day. Just picking up a saucepan off the stove the wrong way can trigger hours of pain in my wrists.

I avoid certain types of weightlifting exercises that I know trigger those muscles to spasm, but I can still handle a certain amount of chin-ups and push-ups. To be honest, it's very weird. I have to be very careful and thoughtful. If you were watching me in the gym, you wouldn't even know I was avoiding so many things.

But it's all so worth it. Adapt. Improvise. And overcome.

Why your mindset matters most

Exercising with type 1 diabetes (T1D) can feel so complicated that many people simply give up. If that's ever been you, I don't blame you. Trying to jog for 30 minutes only to guzzle carbs after 20 minutes to keep yourself alive isn't fun.

Those scary (and obnoxious) lows can drive you to inhale more calories than you tried to burn. On the other hand, the wildly dramatic spikes are especially frustrating and often confusing! Why the heck is your blood sugar spiking when your heart is pounding and you're working so hard?

But it *is* possible to exercise safely and successfully with T1D. It is possible to actually enjoy it, too. This book will teach you what your body needs for different types of exercise, how to simplify your plan for exercise, and how to prevent those frustrating blood sugar fluctuations.

The people you've heard about who successfully exercise with this disease aren't magically special or gifted or luckier than you — they've simply put in the work to learn about the many variables that affect their blood sugar during exercise.

And they don't get it perfectly *all the time*, either. It's easy to get the timing of insulin, carbs, and exercise wrong even with the best intentions and plenty of knowledge.

There is logic to it. There are actual facts about exercise and insulin that *everyone* and *anyone* can learn in order to make exercising with T1D significantly easier and safer.

It does take some work. It requires a variety of "experiments" and being willing to say, "Okay, that didn't work, let's try again." It requires a mindset and an attitude that leaves self-pity at the door.

There is no magic bullet. Despite the fancy technology available today, you still have to learn, plan, and adjust to prevent your blood sugar from plummeting or spiking during even the most casual types of exercise.

We have two choices

We truly have two choices in T1D when it comes to exercise: get frustrated and quit *or* be patient and learn.

That's what we've gotta do as people with T1D. We've got to adapt to the circumstances that affect our blood sugar, improvise a plan to help manage those variables, and overcome the challenges T1D presents.

If you've ever been told that you can't do X, Y, Z because of this disease, you're not alone.

I've heard of doctors telling people they can't go kayaking anymore after their diagnosis, and that they should only go for short walks from now on. My friend was told she certainly couldn't go for long jogs let alone compete in triathlons. (Guess what? She does anyway! Many times!)

But the people who tell us we *can't* are simply very wrong.

What's even *more* important, though, is what you believe. Exercising with T1D is not easy. And even when you learn all that fancy schmancy science, you're still gonna have workouts that don't go smoothly.

Whether you're in the early stages of learning how to exercise with T1D or you've been doing it for years, the ability to say, "Okay, *that* didn't work the way I hoped it would. What can I tweak next time to get different results?"

This problem-solving mindset is *critical* because there are so many variables that can affect your blood sugar before, during, and after exercise. Any person with T1D who has ever exercised safely and successfully — in their neighborhood or in the Olympics or in a reality fitness TV show — has simply mastered one thing: this problem-solving mindset.

Throughout this book, I will be asking you to step back and look at the circumstances surrounding your past experience with exercise and apply new learning to your future exercise endeavors.

The science of what your body wants during exercise is truly the same for every human being. Then, the next step is learning how to mix and mash T1D into that science.

Ready? Here we go!

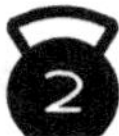

Before you start sweating

Before we dive into the nitty gritty details, let's make sure we're all on the same page about a few very crucial details — the last lengthy bit is the most important!

I am not a doctor — and I am definitely not *your* doctor.

Please talk with your healthcare team before making any changes to your insulin doses or diabetes management regimen.

Exercising with T1D is about managing insulin-on-board (IOB).

This book will teach you about IOB in great detail. Whatever blood fluctuation you experience is basically the result of having too much or too little insulin in your system before, during, or after exercise. The factors contributing to IOB during exercise can be learned, managed, and adjusted! *That* is what this book is all about.

If you're new to exercise after months or years of very little exercise...

The impact of exercise on your daily insulin needs is an awesome thing and you'll see the evidence of this very quickly! The newer you are to exercise, the bigger impact you're going to see in your insulin needs.

You may need an immediate and significant reduction in *all* of your basal/background insulin dose(s) within a day or two of starting a daily exercise routine. You could potentially see your basal/background insulin needs cut by 25 to 50 percent. If you don't make these changes, you'll likely find yourself frustrated and exhausted with recurring low blood sugars.

If you use a closed-loop pump...

Closed-loop pumps are insulin pumps that communicate directly with your continuous glucose monitor (CGM) and automatically make adjustments in your insulin dosages in an effort to prevent fluctuations. While the guidance in this book can be applied to diabetes management with a closed-loop pump, it will not dig into every type of closed-loop system.

The nuts and bolts are the same: you switch to "exercise mode" or "sleep mode," which tells the pump to be less aggressive in its dosing. Some people prefer to switch their pump to "manual mode" to gain full control over all insulin dosing during exercise — and then apply the ideas offered in this book. Whatever you decide, you are still tasked with the responsibility of managing IOB to prevent lows and highs.

Exercising with high blood sugars...

Intentionally exercising with high blood sugars is actually *not* a great option. And most importantly, it's not your only option! If you've been exercising with intentionally high blood sugars, you're not alone. It's extremely common because it feels like the only way to prevent lows.

But your biggest goal as a person with T1D is to stay in your target blood sugar range. Intentionally exercising with high blood sugar is not only dangerous for your long-term health but also dangerous in the short-term, too.

When your blood sugar is over 300 mg/dL...

Please know that this book does *not* recommend exercising when your blood sugar is over 300 mg/dL. Throughout this book, any reference to exercising with high blood sugar does so with the understanding that your blood sugar is below 300 mg/dL.

Exercising with blood sugars over 300 mg/dL can increase your risk of developing ketones and put your body under a great deal of stress. It is up to you and your healthcare team to determine when it is or isn't safe to exercise with blood sugars over 300 mg/dL.

If your blood sugar is over 300 mg/dL, check for ketones using urine/ blood test strips and follow your usual protocol to safely correct the high.

Your basal/background insulin dose(s) probably need fine-tuning.

Before you even add exercise to your diabetes science experiment, we've got some fine-tuning to do. No amount of exercise knowledge will work if your basal/background insulin doses are not accurate.

Nothing will go as planned if you are getting way too much or way too little basal insulin. In fact, even if you are getting just a *tiny bit* too much or too little basal insulin, you'll find yourself quite frustrated during the mildest physical activity!

What I'm *not* going to do in this book is take you through every step of "basal rate testing". Instead, I highly encourage you to read one of the following for the textbook lesson on testing the accuracy of your basal/background insulin:

- **Think Like a Pancreas** by Gary Scheiner, CDCES
- **Pregnancy with Type 1 Diabetes** by Ginger Vieira and Jennifer Smith, RD, CDCES
- **Basal Testing Basics at IntegratedDiabetes.com/basal-testing** by Gary Scheiner CDCES

Chances are that your basal rates need a bit of fine-tuning because your background insulin needs never stick in one place for years on end. They can shift a little throughout any given month or a lot over the course of months and years.

Too often, our healthcare team determines our basal/background insulin dose — then it sits at that number forever. Whether you are pumping or on multiple daily injections, you need to take a close look at your insulin doses regularly. Tiny adjustments by just a few units can have a huge impact on your ability to stay in your goal range whether you're sleeping, working, or jogging.

 **Ginger's example**

Even with 9 units as my current dosage, I still adjust my dose up or down by 1-2 units at times based on variables like my menstrual cycle, slight weight gain, really indulgent meals (pizza, cake, etc.), sudden stressful moments (like adopting a new dog), or the night before Thanksgiving day.

Over the course of *years*, my background insulin dose has changed a lot as my lifestyle habits, age, and body composition changed, too. Here's a look at how much my background insulin dose has changed over the last 15 years:

- **At 20 years old — 32 units total basal insulin:** very sedentary, 150 lbs., poor nutrition habits, regularly overeating

- **At 22 years old — 18 units total basal insulin:** very active teaching yoga/competing in powerlifting, 155 lbs. but now extremely muscular and winning powerlifting competitions, very structured moderate-carb diet

- **At 28 years old — 17 units total basal insulin:** preparing for pregnancy, 128 lbs., thoughtful whole-food diet including some carbs/dessert, etc., very active with low-impact cardio (a lot of dog walks), no longer doing heavy weightlifting

- **At 30 years old — 11 units total basal insulin:** very active, daily cardio exercise, light weightlifting, 125 pounds, busy mother of two, flexible diet with whole foods and regular carbs

- **At 32 years old — increased from 11 units to 16 units total basal insulin nearly overnight:** very active with daily cardio and light weights, 120 lbs., highly stressed for several months while managing the process of divorce with two small children, go go go

- **At 36 years old — 10 units total basal insulin:** very active (mostly jogging or jumping rope and dog walks), 122 lbs., eating my flexible whole-foods diet (including dessert) per usual

- **Weird transition year:** My basal insulin needs kept rising, and with each unit increase, I'd gain another pound. I was very frustrated because there was no reason for it and I felt that my lifestyle habits were certainly disciplined enough to manage my weight. I talked to my endocrinologist about this and discovered many type 1s are taking a GLP-1 medication like Ozempic or Trulicity to manage insulin resistance. (More on this in Chapter 7!)

- **At 37 years old — 9 units total basal insulin:** 115 lbs. I'm doing exactly the same as my 122 lbs. habits but I started taking metformin and semaglutide (Ozempic).

Can you imagine if I'd kept the same background insulin dose over the course of all these years? The big changes in doses came gradually as my body changed from a sedentary body to a powerlifter body to a light weights/cardio exercise body. If I hadn't made these changes, I'd probably be struggling with extreme blood sugar fluctuations and quite miserable!

Little adjustments make a difference!

Whether you use a pump or take insulin via injections/inhalations, little adjustments in your insulin doses are extremely important. The smallest changes in life can require changes in your basal/background insulin needs.

Changes like:

- Losing or gaining even just 5 pounds
- Starting a new habit of walking every day after lunch
- Joining a gym and lifting weights 3 days a week
- Reducing your alcohol consumption
- Starting a new medication
- Quitting smoking
- Going through a divorce
- Starting a new job
- Losing a loved one
- Menstrual cycle starting/ending
- Ovulation, menopause, pregnancy, etc.
- Puberty
- Transitioning to college life
- End of school transition to summer
- Back to school
- Holidays and food-focused celebrations
- Yada, yada, yada!

The list goes on and on.

You may only need an increased/decreased dose for a few days or a few weeks! But that tiny adjustment can make life *so much* easier when your sanity and overall health rely heavily on your ability to manage your blood sugar all day long. Learning how to make these tiny adjustments yourself *at home* is pretty critical. You cannot wait three or six months before your next appointment. Reach out and get support from your healthcare team, but in the meantime, they should also be teaching you how to make adjustments on your own.

I've heard from so many people over the years who have reached out because they're experiencing frequent dramatic swings in their blood sugar levels. One gal had called 911 three times in six months due to sudden severe hypoglycemia — and her doctor *didn't* adjust her background insulin. This young woman was taking 30 units of long-acting insulin every night when she eventually determined that she only needed 20 units.

Another woman who reached out to me was in her 60s and very active, but her new endocrinologist had suddenly told her to increase her long-acting insulin dose by *10 units*. She followed his instructions and was experiencing scary hypoglycemia every afternoon during her routine 6-mile walk. Guzzling juice and candy, trying to save her own life was exhausting. Eventually, she reduced her basal dose back down and was able to enjoy those long walks again. (And yes, she got a new endocrinologist, too.)

These are dramatic examples of getting too much insulin, but even a few units more than you need can wreak havoc on your ability to exercise with T1D. That is the power of insulin!

On the flip side, getting too little background insulin can lead to constant stubborn highs, followed by constant corrections...which leads to constant lows. An exhausting game of T1D yo-yo.

This means you need to pinpoint which came first: the highs or the lows?

Frequent stubborn highs mean you likely need a small boost in your basal. Frequent illogical lows mean you likely need a small decrease (at least) in your basal.

This is a wild simplification of basal testing — I realize — but I also know most people *aren't* going to perform basal testing.

You're probably getting too much basal insulin if you:

- ...go low during a 1-mile walk without any rapid-acting insulin-on-board.

- ...go low during 30 minutes of weightlifting without any rapid-acting insulin-on-board.

- ...go low every single day despite careful meal dosing and you can't figure out why.

- ...feel like anything and everything can cause you to go low.

You probably need *more* basal insulin if you:

- ...are usually high 3 to 4 hours after eating.

- ...often can't correct a high blood sugar within 4 hours.

- ...generally feel like your mealtime/correction insulin "isn't working".

When making adjustments in your basal/background insulin dose(s), it's important to start small. Never make an adjustment of more than 1 to 3 units at a time. If you're more sensitive to insulin, a 1-unit increase/decrease is plenty. If you're more resistant, a 3-unit increase/decrease may be more appropriate.

Then, let that new dose prove itself for 2 to 3 days before making any further decisions — unless it is glaringly obvious that it is too much or too little.

The bigger message is: don't be afraid to make small, thoughtful adjustments to your background insulin. *Small* and *thoughtful* adjustments. You cannot wait until your next appointment 6 months from now to make those tweaks. It's just too long to wait.

And actually, it's dangerous to wait. If you're not getting the right amount of insulin, your health is suffering. And there are just too many reasons our body needs small adjustments to our insulin doses *all the time*.

Thriving with T1D includes learning how to carefully make small adjustments on your own. Period.

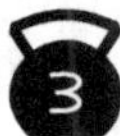

Is your workout aerobic or anaerobic?

There's a big difference between aerobic and anaerobic exercise — especially if you have type 1 diabetes — and we're going to dig into both in this chapter. Knowing the difference between aerobic and anaerobic exercise means knowing how to manage your blood sugar.

Once upon a time, we were taught to simply eat "15 grams of carbohydrate" before any type of exercise, check our blood sugars often, and eat more carbs as needed.

There are a couple of huge problems with this outdated advice:

1. This advice doesn't acknowledge the differences in how aerobic versus anaerobic exercise impact blood sugar levels.

2. This advice doesn't acknowledge "insulin-on-board" (IOB), which plays a big role in how likely your blood sugar will drop.

Here, we're going to look at issue #1: the differences between aerobic versus anaerobic exercise. (Later, we'll talk about all that IOB!)

Aerobic exercise: burn, baby, burn

Examples of aerobic exercise

Walking, jogging, kayaking, rollerblading, power yoga, skating, vacuuming, gardening, cycling, dancing, hiking, chasing kids, etc.

Fancy definition

Aerobic metabolism takes place in the mitochondria of the cell and is able to use carbohydrates, protein, or fat as fuel sources.

Ginger's definition

Aerobic exercise is an activity you can perform for an extended period of time without stopping. During aerobic exercise, your heart rate is still low enough that your body is able to cycle oxygen to your fat cells to burn for fuel. Or, if there's plenty of IOB, your source of fuel will likely be the glucose in your bloodstream.

Aerobic exercise actually increases how quickly insulin picks up glucose and carries it to cells — because your cells are demanding more glucose to keep your body moving and performing!

Naturally, the human body would dramatically reduce insulin production to prevent low blood sugar. Of course, as a person with T1D, that whole system is squashed. This means aerobic exercise can cause fast, dramatic drops in your blood sugar *if you have enough insulin on board.*

You can actually significantly reduce how much glucose aerobic exercise uses for fuel by carefully timing your workouts to avoid excess insulin on board — we'll discuss this more soon!

Anaerobic exercise: a different kind of burn

Examples of anaerobic exercise

Weightlifting, sprints, CrossFit, HIIT workouts, spinning intervals, etc.

Fancy definition

Anaerobic metabolism uses stored glucose (glycogen) from your muscle tissue and your liver as its only source of fuel and produces pyruvate and lactic acid.

Ginger's definition

Anaerobic exercise is an activity that's usually performed at an intensity you can only sustain for a few minutes at most. Then you take a break — for anywhere from 30 seconds to 2 minutes — then you perform another round, and so on.

Your heart rate during anaerobic exercise is so high that your body must use glucose for fuel by converting stored glucose (glycogen) in your muscle tissue and lactic acid to glucose. That glucose is then cycled back to your muscles for fuel with a little help from *insulin*. For some types of anaerobic exercise, the insulin from your basal rate/dose might be plenty. For more intense anaerobic exercise, you may actually need more insulin to manage that extra glucose. (We'll talk about this *a lot*, I promise.)

After anaerobic exercise, your liver might release stored glucose from your liver to help replenish the glucose stores in your muscles — with a little help from *insulin*.

Of course, if you have T1D, you're not producing the insulin needed to manage that extra glucose. This means anaerobic exercise can easily lead to high blood sugars during or after your workout.

What about adrenaline?

Adrenaline-inducing competition can be very tricky! Many people think adrenaline is what spikes blood sugar levels during weightlifting at the gym, but adrenaline is a true fight-or-flight response in true competition.

That soccer *game* can spike your blood sugar 100 points even though you'd normally drop 100 points during practice because of the innate biological response to true competition.

It's hard to prepare for, too, because you can't always predict when that adrenaline might hit. The safest bet is to react after it happens but that can mean you're stuck with a high blood sugar for the rest of the event! So tedious.

As you get more practice with these adrenaline-inducing activities, you can develop a more preventative approach by increasing basal insulin or taking a small bolus at the start of the event. Just remember: low blood sugars ruin *all the fun*, so treat cautiously when dosing here.

When aerobic and anaerobic exercise get easily mixed up

This can all be quite confusing when you feel like your heart is pumping during a weightlifting workout and you're breathing hard — surely your blood sugar ought to be dropping, right? But understanding the science behind these two categories of exercise is critical to exercising safely.

Some types of aerobic exercise can actually become anaerobic — and vice versa. Here are a few examples to keep in mind when trying to predict your workout's impact on your blood sugar.

When aerobic exercise turns anaerobic:

- **Intense sprinting within a regular jog:** Even just a couple rounds of intense sprints within your otherwise casual jog can trigger that anaerobic conversion of stored glycogen into glucose.

- **Short bursts of competitive exercise:** Karate *class* might be steady-state aerobic exercise but rounds of karate *sparring* can be so intense at only 90-seconds long that you easily trigger an anaerobic response. If you're performing any aerobic exercise at an intensity you can only sustain for a few minutes, you can expect your blood sugar to spike.

 **Ginger's example:** I have a 1.7-mile loop that I run several times a week. Every now and then, I feel a little guilty about how short it is (but long runs aren't good for me) and then I try to run it really fast to compensate. During the last half of this 20-minute run, I'm pushing at an intensity that is really quite stressful — in a fun, rigorous sort of way. The last bit of the run includes a lengthy hill and charging up that hill pushes me to the point of gasping for breath at the end. Inevitably, I push myself into a far more *anaerobic* zone and my blood sugar spikes wildly in the last few minutes of my run. That spike continues after I've finished, and the best I can do is respond quickly with a bolus of insulin — since my initial plan was to go for a steady 1.7 jog, not a long sprint! Since there is a delay between my actual blood sugar level and the number on my CGM (which is really measuring glucose in the interstitial fluid in my fat tissue), the spike seems to arrive *after* the workout, but it's mostly like during *and* after.

Anytime you're performing a typical aerobic exercise at an intensity you can only maintain for only a few minutes, you're pushing your body into that anaerobic zone! Take good notes and be consistent to help you better anticipate the impact on your blood sugar.

When anaerobic exercise turns aerobic:

- **Spinning:** Spinning can include a lot of intense bursts of intensity that typically qualify it for an aerobic label. However, if you're spinning at a generally consistent intensity for the entire workout — *without* those super intense bursts — you can easily burn up glucose as described in aerobic exercise.

- **Steady intervals:** If you're simply switching between two minutes of walking and two minutes of jogging, this is likely keeping you in an aerobic state. You're just performing aerobic exercise at different intensities but neither of those intensities is *so intense* that it qualifies as anaerobic.

 **Ginger's example:** I love jumping rope. During the last year or so of my marriage, jumping rope became my therapy and my safe outlet for my stress, energy, and enthusiasm for life! I gradually worked my way up to being able to jump rope nearly non-stop for a full hour. While this hour was a steady jog-like intensity — and thus clearly aerobic — jumping rope can also be *anaerobic* if you want it to be. Many people mix short bursts of jumping rope into a circuit of other anaerobic exercises like weightlifting or sprinting. For me, jumping rope *never* spikes my blood sugar because I prefer to perform it as a moderately steady and lengthy aerobic activity. This means I plan my blood sugar according to aerobic exercise guidelines and expect jumping rope to burn glucose and lower my blood sugar.

Anytime you're performing a typically anaerobic exercise with too much insulin on board, you can easily burn up more glucose as though it's an aerobic workout!

Okay, now we need to take a look at IOB because this is the true factor that can send your blood sugar plummeting during any type of physical activity.

Insulin-on-board matters most

Your IOB matters, baby! It matters big time. Actually, the real secret to exercising with type 1 diabetes comes down to this: managing your insulin-on-board (IOB) and the timing of your workout.

When you have too much IOB within the hours of your workout, your risk of low blood sugar is extremely likely.

There are three common approaches to managing IOB to prevent low blood sugar during exercise:

- Exercising several hours after eating or taking insulin for a meal

- Exercising right after eating but reducing your meal bolus and/or basal insulin

- Exercising when you feel like it and consuming a lot of candy or juice to get through it

First, we'll look at my personal favorite approach: Timing your exercise for several hours since your last meal and insulin bolus — also known as "fasted" exercise. Even if you're fond of this idea, I encourage you to read this section to better grasp how timing, insulin, food, and other factors impact your blood sugar during exercise.

Using "fasted" exercise prevents lows

If you can time your workouts for when you have the least amount of rapid-acting insulin in your system (your IOB), you can hugely reduce your risk of low blood sugar.

In the context of type 1 diabetes, the phrase "fasted" exercise refers to exercising at least several hours after the last time you ate and took mealtime insulin. By exercising *before* you eat a meal, you are exercising when you don't have a large bolus of rapid-acting insulin in your bloodstream.

Fasted exercise is *not* intended for endurance sports — hours of exercising — because your body is obviously going to need re-fueling eventually for long athletic events.

Fasted exercise is ideal for regular ol' workouts, jogs, bike rides, etc. that are no longer than two hours.

And best of all, you can create that fasted environment at *any* time of day — but we're going to start with fasted exercise in the morning.

Please read this paragraph carefully: "Fasted" exercise still requires basal/background insulin — even if it is a significantly reduced dose via your insulin pump. If you're on long-acting injected basal insulin, you may need to make gradual reductions to the daily dose when you add exercise to your routine. As people living with type 1 diabetes, we need *some* active insulin present at all times in order to stay alive. Without enough basal/background insulin at any given time, a person with type 1 diabetes can quickly go into diabetic ketoacidosis — which is extremely dangerous and can be fatal.

So, what the heck is "fasted" exercise?

Creating this fasted environment does *not* mean you have to skip meals or starve yourself. Instead, it just means you're timing your exercise when:

...it's been at least 3 to 4 hours since your last dose of rapid-acting liquid insulin.

- **Injected or pumped insulin:** If you take a bolus of rapid-acting insulin (Novolog, Humalog, Fiasp, etc.) via injection or pump, that insulin is most active in your bloodstream for about 3 to 4 hours. If you exercise during that 4-hour window, your risk of going low is significantly likely. If you can time your workout to take place *after* that 3 to 4-hour window, you can hugely reduce your risk of hypoglycemia.

- **If you use an insulin pump:** You will likely need to reduce your basal rates significantly before aerobic exercise to prevent hypoglycemia. We'll discuss this in great detail later.

...it's been at least 60 to 90 minutes since your last dose of ultra-rapid inhaled insulin.

- **Inhaled insulin:** If you use inhaled insulin for your meals or corrections, that insulin is most active in your bloodstream for 60 to 90 minutes. Exercising during that time frame increases your risk of going low.

Why? Because the less rapid-acting insulin you have active in your bloodstream, the less glucose is going to be rapidly used for fuel.

Fasted exercise forces your body to work a bit harder and burn more fat for fuel instead of that readily available glucose. Your muscles can take up glucose to use for fuel even without insulin present, but IOB can cause them to use significantly more glucose, leading to lows. When you don't have a big bolus of IOB to grab glucose easily for fuel, your muscles use less glucose and burn far more fat for fuel.

When you take a dose of rapid-acting insulin for a meal, your body will burn glucose primarily for fuel while you exercise. Exercise increases the speed at which your cells take up glucose with help from insulin, increasing your risk of hypoglycemia.

As long as your basal/background insulin dose is accurate, you should be able to walk on an empty stomach first thing in the morning *without* experiencing hypoglycemia.

You need to know about dawn phenomenon...

Since we're talking about potentially exercising first thing in the morning, you need to know about dawn phenomenon.

Dawn phenomenon is a term to describe the early morning hormones and neurotransmitters the human body produces to get you going for the day — often affecting your blood sugar the moment your feet hit the floor in the morning! It includes cortisol, growth hormone, epinephrine, and dopamine.

These four troublemakers essentially create insulin resistance and tell your liver to release stored sugar (glycogen) and convert it to glucose (sugar).

This can look like a small, medium, or large spike in your blood sugar. (Over-eating (or binge-eating) before bed can make dawn phenomenon more dramatic because your body still dealing with that abundance of calories and carbohydrates.)

Some people experience that dawn phenomenon spike the moment their feet hit the floor in the morning. Others find it's more about time than being awake. If you eat breakfast quickly after waking up, you may not notice or experience dawn phenomenon because you're already giving your brain fuel through nutrition instead of glucose from your liver.

- **If you use a pump:** You can adjust your basal settings to anticipate and target this early morning spike. Remember, your basal settings between 4 and 5 a.m. are really what affect your blood sugar between 5 and 6 a.m., so adjustments need to be made in anticipation of dawn phenomenon, not during the exact hour you see that spike.

- **If you take injections:** You may find you simply need to take a small bolus of rapid-acting insulin as soon as you wake up. You might be able to increase your long-acting insulin dose but it may cause lows at other times of day even if it is the amount you need to prevent dawn phenomenon spikes. A tricky balancing act!

- **If you use inhaled insulin:** Inhaled insulin is really *too* fast (and out too fast) to properly manage the gradual spike caused by dawn phenomenon. Ideally, you'd supplement your inhaled insulin regimen with a small injection of rapid-acting for circumstances like this.

 **Ginger's example**

- **Most mornings these days, I wake up at 5:30 a.m.** to squeeze in 30 minutes of jumping rope before my kids wake up. I simply know my body and my brain feel so ready for the day when I make those 30 minutes a priority. Then I get my kids to school and take my dog for a 40-minute walk. This *doesn't* drop my blood sugar because my body is still in fasting mode and I haven't taken a large bolus of insulin for food — instead, my blood sugar is far more likely to rise due to dawn phenomenon.

- **I used to experience a 100-point spike in my blood sugar** between 6:30 to 7:30 a.m.—and I'd need at least a ¼ or ½ unit of rapid-acting injected insulin to manage that spike *while* also jumping rope. (Since I don't like pens or pumps, I'd stick a syringe into the pen as though it is a vial and eyeball a ¼ unit smidge of insulin.)

- **These days, I've been taking 1,000 mg of metformin (a medication usually prescribed for type 2 diabetes)** before bed and once-weekly semaglutide (a GLP-1 medication) — more on this in Chapter 7! These medications actually suppress that dawn phenomenon surge of glucose from my liver! If I continue to fast past 8 a.m., I still need a very small dose of rapid-acting insulin, but the spike from dawn phenomenon is significantly smaller, happens about an hour later, and is easier to manage.

- **Read more about my experience with metformin and semaglutide to manage dawn phenomenon here:** T1Dexchange.org/semaglutide-type-1-diabetes

If you're going to perform fasted exercise in the morning, you'll need to pinpoint whether dawn phenomenon is a factor you need to plan for. Many people with T1D experience dawn phenomenon but there's certainly some who don't.

Your basal/background insulin doses must be fine-tuned

If you're getting too much or too little basal/background insulin via injected long-acting insulin or pumped rapid-acting insulin, fasted exercise simply ain't gonna go as planned. Learning how to fine-tune and adjust your background dose(s) is a must.

Please keep in mind that adjustments to your basal/background insulin doses should be done in very small tweaks — a change of no more than 1 or 2 units total at a time for insulin-sensitive to people. For those on larger doses, your doctor may recommend larger adjustments of 3+ units at a time.. Watch the impact for a couple days, then adjust again if needed.

Here are the basics to consider when fine-tuning background insulin doses for fasted exercise:

Low blood sugars during fasted exercise likely mean: You are getting too much basal/background insulin whether it's aerobic or anaerobic.

- **If you're on injected long-acting insulin:** Sometimes a tiny adjustment can make a huge difference. A reduction of just 1 or 2 units can address those lows, but don't be surprised if that means you need a bit more for meals. It's all a big balancing act. That excess long-acting insulin may have been covering more of your mealtime insulin needs than necessary. The goal is to never be "feeding your insulin," which means you should be able to go for a walk without mealtime insulin in your system and not go low.

  - I have met a few people who were taking 10 more units of long-acting a day than they needed thanks to haphazard adjustments by their doctor. Their lows were frequent and dramatic. Take a closer look at how often you're experiencing low blood sugars. Frequent severe low blood sugars mean you are getting way too much basal/background insulin — plus it's simply dangerous!

- **If you are on an insulin pump:** Most people find they need to reduce basal rates by anywhere from 25 to 75 percent starting 1 hour before aerobic exercise. It certainly requires a great deal of trial and error — and we'll discuss it further in this book in more detail. Most people also have already adjusted their basal rates to account for spikes in the early morning due to dawn phenomenon, so that is less of a factor to consider if you're pumping.

High blood sugars during fasted exercise likely mean: You're not getting enough insulin either via basal/background OR you need a small bolus to address spikes caused by anaerobic exercise or dawn phenomenon.

- **How do you know which insulin dose needs tweaking?** If you don't see a rise in your blood sugar during that same time frame when you're *not* exercising (or eating), the cause of your high is likely related to the effects of your exercise or dawn phenomenon if you're on injections. This means you likely need a very small bolus of rapid-acting insulin right before or during your workout. (Sometimes a ½ is more than enough when you combine it with exercise!) Remember, if you perform an aerobic workout during that same time frame, you may not need that bolus! These little details matter. Take notes and control as many factors as possible to create consistency between experiments!

The tiniest adjustments can make a big difference! Just 1 or 2 units added or subtracted from your total basal/background insulin dose(s) can make it that much easier to enjoy exercise safely.

Wait, what about coffee?!?!?

If you need that morning coffee before you start working out, you're not alone. Some people experience a noteworthy rise in blood sugar due to caffeine. Caffeine essentially does the same thing that dawn phenomenon hormones do: triggers your liver to release stored sugar to give you a boost of energy.

Some people need a small dose of insulin with that coffee — even without adding cream or sugar. Simply put, the more you complicate your coffee with additional ingredients, the more complicated your morning exercise regimen will be.

 ## Ginger's example

- **Fasted exercise inspired me to stop putting cream or artificial sweeteners in my coffee.** Cold-turkey, I started drinking my coffee completely black. It tasted truly terrible for the first month. Then my taste buds were reborn — and I could actually appreciate the flavor of coffee without dressing it up like a dessert. My taste buds no longer care for the sweetened version of coffee. I highly recommend experimenting with training your taste buds to enjoy plain black coffee! It tastes delicious — eventually!

- **When it comes to its impact on my diabetes,** I know that one cup of coffee does not spike my blood sugar at all. If I drink another cup, my blood sugar spikes over 250 mg/dL and won't come down for hours until the caffeine has cleared my system. Even decaf coffee causes this spike! So what do I do? I limit myself to one cup of coffee and switch to caffeine-free tea if I still want another hot beverage.

I know, coffee is precious. I hear you. But excessive amounts of caffeine can also hugely contribute to insulin resistance, weight gain, anxiety, and difficulty sleeping! The more caffeine you consume throughout the day, the more likely you're needing higher amounts of basal/background insulin which can also lead to weight-gain. Getting a handle on your caffeine consumption can be hugely beneficial to your diabetes management. (The FDA recommends no more than four cups of coffee a day! As people with diabetes, we should definitely consider the impact its having on our blood sugars and insulin resistance.)

What about a really low-carb meal?

Sure! If you can eat a few cubes of cheese and some cucumber without needing a bolus of insulin, you could get away with a small snack before fasted exercise. In reality, protein and fat *do* raise blood sugar eventually, so this could be a tricky game to play. But if you need to eat a lil' something, a small low-carb meal would be your best bet — perhaps 15 grams of carbohydrates or less to minimize the amount of insulin you need to take.

Fasted exercise does NOT have to happen in the morning

Okay, back to fasting: Yes, you can create a fasted environment at *any* time of day! It really comes down to timing your workouts properly to reduce the amount of rapid-acting IOB.

 **Ginger's examples**

- **I plan to go to karate class at 6 p.m. tonight** — literally two hours from the moment I first typed this sentence. I anticipate karate being more aerobic than anaerobic and hope to have as little as possible mealtime insulin in my system by the start of class. My last meal was around 2:30 p.m. I made a slow-digesting protein shake (frozen strawberries, 1 scoop of Orgain Simple protein powder, a big blob of peanut butter, and unsweetened almond milk). I knew I had to get this slow-digesting meal in my belly before 3 p.m. I used a combination of injected and inhaled insulin to cover this meal. While I only took 2 units of Novolog, I personally still want *at least* 3 hours between that dose and karate class. This will hugely reduce my risk of going low during class. Others might be able to get away with exercising within 2 hours of taking a bolus rapid-acting insulin.

- **When my children were babies** — and they woke up at the crack of dawn—my best opportunity for exercise was at 7 p.m. after they'd been put to bed. I made sure my last meal was around 3 p.m. (I didn't use inhaled insulin back then.) If I couldn't eat until 4 p.m., I would choose a very low-carb snack to ensure I needed a very small bolus of insulin. Once the babies were snoozing, I would jump rope for 45 to 60 minutes *and then eat a late dinner.*

- **A couple of days a week, I visit the gym in the late afternoon** (when I don't have my kids after school) for a steady 2-mile jog and 20 minutes of light weights, likely around 4 or 5 p.m. I plan for this by ensuring that I eat by 1 p.m. if I plan to cover the meal with injected insulin or by 2 p.m. if I plan to use inhaled insulin.

- **This past fall, I coached my daughter's kindergarten soccer team.** Practice and games were every Saturday morning at 10:15 a.m. The last place I want to have a low blood sugar is when I'm responsible for the management of 12 kindergarteners! I never experienced a single low while coaching because I *skipped breakfast* entirely thanks to intermittent fasting. Instead, this meant I could run around freely without lows, but I was more likely going to see a rise in my blood sugar due to fasting beyond 9 a.m. My liver would compensate for skipping breakfast by releasing a wallop of stored sugar and I would take a small bolus of a ½ or 1-unit of injected insulin for this right before practice started. Without that extra little bolus, I would've found myself at 250 mg/dL by 11 a.m. (Learn more about intermittent fasting in Chapter 7!)

- **Every day, I walk my dogs around 12 or 1 p.m.** I prepare my blood sugar for this by simply eating lunch *after* the walk instead of before. If I really wanted to eat lunch before, I could take a significantly reduced bolus for the meal and likely enjoy the 30-minute walk without going low. But it's a lot easier to simply eat lunch after the walk! Now that I use inhaled insulin, I can potentially eat lunch at noon and walk my dogs at 1 p.m. The only tricky detail there is that I might need a "follow-up" dose of inhaled insulin because it clears my system before the meal has been digested. If I know I still have food digesting by 1 p.m., I'll usually go for my walk and keep an eye on my blood sugar. If I see it start to rise, I'll take a small dose of inhaled insulin halfway through the walk and use the combination of the walk and the insulin to prevent any spike from the meal — all while hugely reducing my risk of going low.

- **Keep fast-acting carbs with you to treat lows always!** Just another reminder to keep fast-acting carbs with you *always, always, always* when you're exercising.

What if my blood sugar is low before fasted exercise?

If your blood sugar is low before your planned fasted exercise then *heck*, you need to eat some fast-acting carbs! But the details around your low blood sugar matter big time.

- **If you are low but it's been at least 3 hours since your last bolus of insulin**, you might be able to eat a small amount of carbohydrates (5 to 15 grams depending on the severity of the low) and wait until you're at a safe number before exercising. You should keep a close eye on your blood sugar during your workout to ensure you don't dip low again.

- **If you are low and it's only been 2 hours since your last bolus of insulin**, you are not in a fasted environment. Your risk of going low even *after* treating the low is very likely.

- **If you're stuck in a habit of over-treating low blood sugars**, this is a huge opportunity to nix this self-destructive habit. We'll chat about this more in Chapter 6 or check-out *Emotional Eating with Diabetes* (by Ginger Vieira on Amazon).

What if my blood sugar is high before fasted exercise?

Exercise can be a great way to correct a high blood sugar, but you don't want to crash! And exercising when you're high might prevent lows but it's really not ideal for your health.

The solution? A really tiny dose of correction insulin.

For example:

- **Situation:** Your usual correction factor is 1 unit to drop your blood sugar 25 points, but your blood sugar is 250 mg/dL and you're about to go for a 30-minute jog.

- **Any insulin already on board?** Fasted exercise implies it's been at least 3 to 4 hours since your bolus of insulin, right? Really think about how much IOB might be part of this equation before taking additional correction insulin.

- **Correction dose:** With a correction factor of 1:25, you'd normally take at least 4 hours to get your blood sugar under 150 mg/dL. Taking a correction dose before exercise means you likely need only 25 percent of that correction dose. Start on the side of caution! This means taking 1 unit of rapid-acting insulin to help your blood sugar come down *safely* without crashing.

- **Remember, injected rapid-acting insulin takes 45 minutes to really get going in your system**—which means you shouldn't expect to be down to 100 mg/dL by the end of your 30-minute run.

- **Remember, if you're already taking insulin to correct a high**, you likely don't need additional insulin for dawn phenomenon. If repeated experiments prove that you need more insulin because your blood sugar is still high after your workout, then you can consider taking a large correction dose.

- **The longer your workout is, the more caution you should apply** when taking correction insulin. Sometimes it just takes a tiny smidge (like ¼ unit) of rapid-acting insulin to correct a high during exercise. It all depends on your insulin sensitivity.

- **Even if you're doing anaerobic exercise**, use caution when taking correction insulin before exercise.

 ## Ginger's example

- **If I'm low before fasted exercise, I treat the low with as few carbohydrates as possible.** If I wake up at 5:30 a.m. with a blood sugar of 50 mg/dL, I treat it with only about 5 grams of rapid-acting carbs (1 glucose tab or 3 Skittles or 3 Sour Patch kids, etc.). I know that my dawn phenomenon will kick me up to 120 mg/dL by the time I start jumping rope. I know I don't need more than 5 grams unless I'm severely low and sweating—which would also mean I should skip my morning jump rope workout.

- **Even if the low is midday before a fasted dog walk**, I know that without any mealtime IOB, I don't need very much to treat the low *and* endure the dog walk. Of course, I still carry a bunch of fast-acting carbs with me, just in case. But I rarely need more than those simple 5 grams.

- **I don't panic.** I remind myself that I'm capable of treating this low. I consider the variables at play — insulin, dawn phenomenon, carbs — and I treat the low with as few carbohydrates as possible to avoid going high during my exercise.

What if I have correction IOB from a high blood sugar earlier in the day?

So you took insulin to correct a high blood sugar at 2 p.m. but you want to exercise at 4 p.m.?

- **Aerobic exercise:** You may need to eat a small amount of carbs to compensate for that IOB. If it's been 2 hours or less since taking that correction dose, chances are you could go low during aerobic exercise without additional carbohydrates. The bigger the correction dose was, the more carbs you might need to eat.

- **Anaerobic exercise:** If you're about to do a workout that normally spikes your blood sugar, that leftover correction dose might be your best friend and prevent you from needing additional insulin before/during your workout.

You could also allow your fasted exercise goals to inspire you to be very cautious when dosing correction insulin. We all get frustrated with highs and have to fight the urge to "rage bolus" and take a big correction in the hope that it'll come down sooner. (Hint: Taking more insulin doesn't make it act faster!) Resist that urge to rage bolus so you don't disrupt your exercise plans a few hours later.

Fasted exercise isn't for everyone

Fasted exercise isn't for everyone. Maybe you don't want to plan that much ahead or you like snacking all day long or you just don't feel good exercising on an empty stomach. That's okay!

You can still keep fasted exercise in mind when you need to plan for something out of your usual routine filled with unknowns — like a company hike or taking your kids to the playground. Knowing you don't have a bolus of insulin in your system can relieve some anxiety and allow you to enjoy the moment.

Regardless of whether you exercise fasted or not, learning how to master the timing of insulin vs. exercise is the true ticket to enjoying exercise without crazy blood sugar fluctuations.

Exercising right after eating a meal

Okay, you'd like to exercise shortly after eating? It's possible! In some ways, it's more complicated than fasted exercise because you have the massive variables of food and insulin to consider. But it's simpler in other ways because it allows you to be more flexible with the timing of your exercise.

Let's take a closer look.

Keep it simple

The easiest way to exercise shortly after eating is to at least be consistent with *what* you're eating. The more familiar you are with how that meal impacts your blood sugar and how much insulin you normally need to cover it, the easier it will be to adjust for exercise.

In other words: eating pizza right before your plan to run a 5K is going to make that 5K a lot more complicated. (Save the pizza for *after* your workout!)

But it comes down to identifying whether you're doing aerobic or anaerobic exercise, too.

- **Aerobic exercise:** You'll absolutely need to reduce your meal bolus by 25 to 90 percent depending on the intensity and duration of your workout. If you're newer to exercising, you'll be more sensitive to the impact of exercise compared to when your body is more conditioned.

  - **If you're on a pump:** You might also need to reduce your basal insulin rate using a "temp basal" starting during the hour *before* you plan to exercise. The reduction percentage can vary wildly (again, anywhere from 25 to 90 percent) and based on the intensity and duration of your workout. Making too many adjustments at one time can be confusing, though, so you may want to start with leaving your basal rate as is and just adjusting your meal bolus. See how that goes, take good notes, and continue tweaking as needed.

- **Anaerobic exercise:** If you know your anaerobic workout tends to spike your blood sugar, you may not need to reduce your meal bolus at all or by only a very small percentage.

  - **If you're on a pump:** The same goes for your basal rates. If you know your anaerobic workout tends to spike your blood sugar, you may not need to reduce your basal rate settings at all or only by a very small percentage.

The easiest way to pinpoint how much insulin is needed for a meal eaten right before exercise is to create consistency by controlling as many factors as you can.

- Time of day
- What you eat
- Type of exercise (aerobic vs. anaerobic)
- Insulin on board (from previous meals & current meal)

Once you've repeated that particular experiment enough times with success in keeping your blood sugar in your target range, you could then be more flexible with what you eat. You have to put in the work, create the experiments, review the results, adjust as needed, and repeat.

 ## Ginger's example

- **In my early 20s, I taught a lot of power yoga classes — definitely aerobic.** (This was before CGMs were available!) I hadn't learned about fasted exercise yet and I definitely had IOB from previously eaten meals. I knew that a 6-ounce strawberry yogurt eaten right before teaching yoga would generally keep my blood sugar between 100 to 200 mg/dL. If I was teaching yoga today, I would absolutely arrange my meals to ensure I was in a fasted environment before class began.

- **In my early 20s, I trained in competitive powerlifting — definitely anaerobic.** Again, no CGMs or knowledge of fasted exercise yet. Instead, I knew these workouts would spike my blood sugar up to 100 points, so I didn't worry about IOB from previously eaten meals and I would usually take 1 unit of rapid-acting insulin *right* before training. Then immediately after, I would eat a small serving of oatmeal with protein powder and water — guzzling it before my next personal training client arrived for their workout! I took a full dose of insulin for that post-workout meal but knew I had to reduce the insulin at my *next* meal when my muscles were really trying to recover.

- **If I'm simply too hungry to do my afternoon dog walk *before* eating lunch,** I know I can cut my meal bolus down by 50 percent for a walk in under 30 minutes — taking a small inhaled insulin dose instead of a medium dose. For a longer walk, I could cut my bolus by 75 percent and take a smidge of rapid-acting injected insulin. If I am just too darn hungry to do my afternoon dog walk before eating lunch, I cut my lunch bolus down by at least 50 percent, if it's just a 15-20 minute walk. If it's going to be another 45-minute walk, I'd cut my lunch bolus down by 75 percent.

There's no magic bullet! There is thoughtful trial and error while trying to manage different variables. Always air on the side of caution and be prepared for lows. It will likely take you many rounds of "experimenting" to learn this balancing act for your body. Take good notes. Take a deep breath. Try again.

What if I want to eat a meal with the least impact on my exercise plans?

Fat and protein are your friends here — and non-starchy vegetables!

Fat and protein *do* affect blood sugar levels, but the impact is so gradual that you could use a low-carb/high-fat or high-protein meal to fill your belly before a workout without needing a wallop of insulin to prevent a big spike.

For example, if you know you'll have a little bit too much IOB during your jog from recent basal or bolus insulin, a spoonful of peanut butter with a handful of raw green pepper slices could gently keep your blood sugar up. Or if you simply want to eat *something* without adding more insulin to the equation, fat and protein-based meals are going to be your simplest bet.

Low-carb/high-protein or high-fat snack examples:
- A handful of cashews and some baby carrots
- Cheese slices and cucumbers
- Cottage cheese and almost
- Raw broccoli and low-carb salad dressing
- Deli meat slices and bell peppers
- Chicken and sautéed onions

You're using the slow-digesting impact of these low-carb but high-protein/fat snacks to blunt the impact of IOB without requiring *more* insulin in order to prevent a super spike.

What if my blood sugar is low before eating and exercising?

Like we discussed in the last chapter: your blood sugar is low before your planned fasted exercise then *yes*, you need to eat some fast-acting carbs! But the details around your low blood sugar matter big time.

- **If you are low and also about to eat a meal before exercising,** this can be a little messy depending on how much IOB is causing your low in the first place. In many cases—especially if there is a lot of IOB — you may need to sit this one out or wait several *hours* instead of minutes. With experience, you might feel comfortable treating the low and IOB with a small meal, waiting until your blood sugar is at a safe level, and exercising as planned. Regardless, you will likely need a more significant reduction in your mealtime insulin if you're starting the meal with a low.

- **If you're stuck in a habit of over-treating low blood sugars,** this is a huge opportunity to nix this self-destructive habit. Learning how to break this habit takes time, but that's really all it is—a habit. A few basic tips to change those habits:

- **Treat lows with foods you've labeled as "medicine" instead of everyday foods** or meals you love. Fast-acting carbohydrates glucose tabs, fat-free gummies or candies, maple syrup, honey, and juice boxes.

- **Stop using lows as an excuse to eat foods you've deemed "off-limits."** Remove the rules! Enjoy those foods in reasonable portions when your blood sugar is in your goal range and you can be thoughtful with how much you eat and how you dose insulin for it.

- **Distract yourself after treating the low until your symptoms calm down.** Try chewing gum, drinking a tall glass of cold water, or noshing some baby carrots until those intense cravings to keep eating pass.

- **Remind yourself, "I am in control of how I treat this low."** It's true. Sure, your brain is begging you to eat more, but you're still in charge of how much food you put in your mouth. Stop giving in to the urge and remind yourself of how much better you'll feel if you are *patient* and treat the low carefully with a thoughtful amount of fast-acting carbohydrates.

- **Read *Emotional Eating with Diabetes*** (by Ginger Vieira on Amazon) for more support in improving your relationship with food as a person with type 1 diabetes.

What if my blood sugar is high before eating and exercising?

Diabetes is so much fun, right? This scenario is a common one and it can feel frustrating, too.

A few things to keep in mind if you're about to eat a meal, your blood sugar is high, and you plan to exercise after eating:

- **Do not rage bolus.** Resist the urge to take a wallop of insulin just because you're high and eat a meal before exercising.

- **Do not take a correction dose in addition to your meal bolus.**

- **You'll likely still need a reduced dose for the meal even though you're already high.** If you usually reduce your meal bolus by 75 percent before exercising, you may only need to reduce it by 50 percent to compensate for the high blood sugar.

- **Be extra thoughtful in what you choose to eat at that meal.** The simpler your meal is, the simpler your ability to exercise and safely correct that high blood sugar will be. This scenario would not be a great time to inhale a few slices of pizza simply because the timing of how pizza digests and the dense carbohydrates and fat it contains will complicate the heck out of your insulin dosing and effort to get back in your target range.

Whether you eat or not, exercising with T1D is always about managing the amount of insulin active in your system at that time. The more consistent and thoughtful you are about what you eat before exercising, the sooner you'll learn what adjustments you need to make to get through it in your goal range.

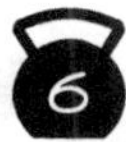

What happens after exercise

You may have finished the workout, but your diabetes work isn't done. Exercise can impact your blood sugar noticeably for up to 12 hours afterward. You might see a milder impact for up to 24 hours after exercise.

Checking your blood sugar *frequently* in the hours after exercising is very important — especially if you're new to that workout and still learning. It wouldn't be overkill to check your blood sugar at least once an hour as you're learning and fine-tuning your insulin doses.

The newer you are to exercising, the more you'll notice that impact across every aspect of your insulin doses — within days of adding exercise to your daily routine. The more you stick to that new habit, the more you'll see your insulin sensitivity increase.

Here, we'll look at when, why, and how exercise impacts your blood sugar after you're done.

Aerobic vs. anaerobic still matters

There are a few differences and a lot of similarities between the post-workout impact of aerobic vs. anaerobic exercise on your blood sugar.

If you did a workout consisting of *both* anaerobic and aerobic exercise then please take *all* of the following guidelines into account.

Please keep in mind that intensity and duration matter here. Walking your dog for 30 minutes is a *great* way to burn calories and body fat, but it probably won't impact your blood sugar for many hours after the walk. That's okay! That keeps life a little simpler.

Similarly, the post-workout impact of a gentler weightlifting session probably won't impact your blood sugar with the same intensity as described below.

These post-workout guidelines apply largely to more intense types of aerobic and anaerobic exercise. Check your blood sugar *often* before, during, and after your workout!

Aerobic exercise: post-workout

- **Reminder: the intensity matters. If you're doing low-intensity cardio like a powerwalk, you won't see as dramatic an impact on your blood sugar in the hours that follow.** However, you'll likely still need a slight reduction in your insulin doses for meals or basal rates during the 4 to 12 hours after your workout.

- **The meal(s) you eat within the next 6 to 12 hours after an intense aerobic workout** will likely need anywhere from 25 to 50 percent less insulin than the amount you'd normally take if you'd been on the couch all day.

- **If you're on long-acting insulin, you can't easily make adjustments** in your basal rate, so reducing your meal bolus doses is likely a must.

- **If you're using a pump, you may also find a temporary reduced basal rate helpful**, anywhere from 10 to 50 percent for up to 12 hours after your workout. But reducing mealtime insulin in addition to reducing your basal rate could be more reductions than necessary. Start with one reduction at a time, take good notes, and make further adjustments as needed.

- **The more consistent you are with exercising regularly**, the more likely you'll be able to make *more permanent* reductions in your basal/background insulin dose(s). This means you'll potentially need to worry less about lows in the hours after exercising. This doesn't mean it always has to be the same type of exercise — any type of daily exercise will help you maintain that sensitivity. Just keep in mind that suddenly going a few days *without* exercise could mean your blood sugars trend a little higher on those days if you don't increase your basal/background dose.

- **The more conditioned your body becomes by exercising several times a week**, the less dramatic the post-workout impact on your blood sugars will be.

- **If you suddenly increase your workout intensity or duration**, the more likely you'll need to further decrease your insulin needs throughout the following 24 hours.

- **Do you need a post-workout meal for aerobic exercise?** Technically, not really to the same severity you would after an anaerobic workout. Sure, you need your *next* meal as planned, but you don't need to specifically eat a meal to recover from aerobic exercise in the same way you would for anaerobic exercise. If your 5K run starts turning into a half-marathon, then *yes*, you would clearly need to pay close attention to your recovery nutrition — but this isn't the book for endurance training!

- **If you exercise in the late afternoon or at night, take extra caution when dosing for meals eaten before bed.** Throughout your snooze, your body is going to be recovering from that workout and your insulin sensitivity will be higher. You might even find you need a small snack before bed *without* a meal bolus OR you need a noticeable reduction in your basal rate as described above. And of course, keep in mind how any adjustments might impact dawn phenomenon the next morning!

Anaerobic exercise: post-workout

- **Reminder: the intensity matters. If you're doing a lighter weightlifting workout**, you likely won't see a dramatic spike in your blood sugar described in this section. However, you'll likely still need a slight reduction in your insulin doses for meals or basal rates during the 4 to 12 hours after your workout.

- **During the hour after a grueling weightlifting or CrossFit workout**, you might notice a rapid spike in your blood sugar. This is likely the result of your liver releasing stored glucose to replenish the sugar stores in your muscle cells and build new muscle.

- **If you don't plan to eat a post-workout meal**, you may still need to take a small bolus of insulin because your muscles do need glucose to replenish their energy stores. Your liver will release stored glycogen, convert it to glucose, and raise your blood sugar if you don't have that extra bolus on board.

- **This is why post-workout meals are important for intense anaerobic workouts.** Your body needs fuel to immediately start the recovery process — which includes building new muscle. (If you weren't aware, you grow new muscle by breaking down your existing muscle through anaerobic exercise which causes it to recover and grow further, in a nutshell.) If you don't fuel your body enough after intense anaerobic exercise, your muscles will struggle to recover and struggle to grow stronger.

- **Ideally, you can avoid that post-workout spike by intentionally eating a small meal** that contains both protein, carbohydrates, and maybe some fat. You'll need insulin for that small meal. This will lessen the need for your liver to release stored glucose. Your body needs this fuel. It doesn't have to be expensive or fancy. It just needs to include some real food. Protein shakes are popular because they are easy and digest quickly, but you can still benefit from eating simple whole foods, too. A few ideas:

    - Protein shake + fruit
    - Protein shake + oats
    - Banana + peanut butter + milk
    - Apple + cheese
    - Apple + veggies + hummus
    - Tuna fish + crackers
    - Cottage cheese + pita bread
    - Yogurt + nuts
    - Eggs + toast
    - Ham slices + cheese + apple

- **Protein powder may look low-carb, but your body does need insulin** to cover large servings of protein. Excess protein is converted into sugar. Don't freak out if your protein powder containing 4 grams of carbohydrates actually impacts your blood sugar and insulin needs like 25 grams of carbs. This is normal. Fine-tune your meal bolus for that protein shake and be consistent in how you prepare it so you can be confident in how many units of insulin to take.

- **Next, you should prepare to need far less insulin at the meal you eat within 4 to 12 hours after your workout.** In other words, if you did CrossFit at 2 p.m. and ate your post-workout meal at 3:30 p.m., you should anticipate needing anywhere from

25 to 75 percent reduction in the meal bolus for your next meal at dinnertime.

- **Your increased insulin sensitivity can last for over 12 hours** as your muscles work to recover from that workout.

- **If you're on long-acting insulin, you can't easily make adjustments in your basal rate**, so reducing your meal bolus doses is likely a must. Some people will reduce their long-acting dose for the day after an intense weightlifting, but that can get messy and hard to remember.

- **If you're using a pump, you may also find a temporary reduced basal rate helpful**, anywhere from 10 to 50 percent for up to 12 hours after your workout. But reducing mealtime insulin in addition to reducing your basal rate could be more reductions than necessary. Start with one reduction at a time, take good notes, and make further adjustments as needed.

- **The more consistent you are with exercising at least every other day**, the more likely you'll be able to make *more permanent reductions* in your basal/background insulin dose(s) and the less you'll need to worry about lows in the hours after exercising. This doesn't mean it always has to be the same type of exercise — any type of daily exercise will help you maintain that sensitivity. When it comes to intense weightlifting or CrossFit, taking days off to let your muscles recover and grow is critical. This means alternating with aerobic exercise is ideal!

- **If you are performing intense heavy weightlifting and *gaining* weight** (via muscle) don't be surprised if your background insulin needs actually increase a bit. That muscle requires more circulating glycogen (converted into glucose) to help grow and maintain that tissue. This isn't a bad thing, it's simply your body growing more tissue that requires more insulin in order to provide it with the fuel it needs.

- **The more conditioned your body becomes by exercising several times a week**, the less dramatic the post-workout impact on your blood sugars will be.

- **If you exercise in the late afternoon or at night, take extra caution when dosing for meals eaten before bed**. Throughout your snooze, your body is going to be recovering from that workout and your insulin sensitivity will be higher. You might even find you need a small snack before bed *without* a meal bolus OR you need a noticeable reduction in your basal rate as described above.

 ## Ginger's examples

- **If I don't jump rope in the morning for whatever reason**, I need nearly twice as much insulin for my lunch of fruit and nuts. For me, the morning jump rope session is the normal day, so the adjustment I have to keep track of is actually taking *more* insulin on the mornings I don't jump rope. But it reveals just how much that morning cardio session is doing for my insulin sensitivity!

- **Today, I will be going to the gym around 5 p.m. to run 2 to 3 miles** and lift very light weights for 20 minutes. Then I'll head home for dinner. I know I'll need half as much insulin for dinner and dessert thanks to this end-of-day workout compared to the days when I only jump rope and walk my dog earlier in the day. I know I'll be more sensitive throughout the night, too, because I'm exercising at the end of the day compared to my morning workout's impact on my daytime meals.

- **Back in my youthful years of competitive powerlifting and personal training**, I quickly learned that *not* eating immediately after a training session would lead to a 100-point spike in my blood sugar. If I couldn't eat right away, I'd need a unit of rapid-acting injected insulin. Normally, I would mix 1 cup of chocolate protein powder with a ½ cup of rolled oats, mix with a little water, eat it quickly, and train my next client. I knew I needed 4 units of rapid-acting insulin for that post-workout meal.

- **The worst low blood sugar I've ever experienced was in my early powerlifting days.** I trained with my coach for an hour around 3 p.m. Then I ate my post-workout meal as described above, trained my own clients until 6 or 7 p.m., then headed home for dinner. But I *forgot* to reduce my insulin dose for that dinner. I took way too much. Within 30 minutes, I noticed my vision starting to go really fuzzy. (Again, there are no CGMs at this time.) I knew I was low, but I couldn't convince myself to stand up. Instead, I crawled over to the kitchen (thankfully, it was a tiny apartment) and pulled a container of oatmeal off the counter. I remember pouring some dry oatmeal into my mouth and trying to chew it. I woke up about an hour later with my face on the carpet. I was okay, but I had clearly lost consciousness for a moment due to severe hypoglycemia. Fortunately, I lived to tell the tale and I've never lost consciousness during a low blood sugar since. (Emergency glucagon would've been helpful here! Unfortunately, I hadn't filled my glucagon prescription.)

- **The other morning, I jumped rope for 60 minutes instead of my usual 30 or 40.** I was watching a great movie and enjoying my jump rope, so I just kept going. A few hours later, I went to a pretty mellow karate class. (Clearly, my kids were with their father this day and I was enjoying my free time.) Well, I had six mild low blood sugars throughout the rest of that day! I completely overlooked how much more work it is for my body to add another 20 minutes of jumping rope. I should've taken reduced doses for most of my meals.

Remember, the first goal is to prevent low blood sugars

Your first goal is to prevent low blood sugars. While I know we all feel terribly guilty seeing high numbers, we also need to air on the side of caution.

- **Recurring lows mean**: you're getting too much insulin
- **Recurring highs mean**: you're not getting enough insulin

Neither of these recurring situations is great for your long-term health and safety.

I know it sounds painfully simple but too often people get mad about the blood sugar fluctuation instead of simply considering these two statements. Stop wasting energy getting mad and simply reflect on the notes of your experiment — then make adjustments. The more consistency you can create in those early experiments, the more you'll learn about what your body needs *after* different types of exercise.

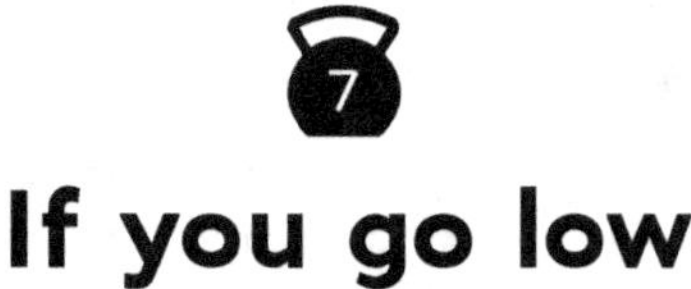

If you go low

Low blood sugars can be really scary. Low blood sugars when you're exercising can be downright terrifying — especially if you're on a dog walk or a jog and you're still a mile from home. (And remember: always bring fast-acting carbs with you no matter what!)

Let's take a closer look at being prepared for lows and managing lows during exercise.

Look at your current habits around treating lows

There's no tip-toeing around it: if you currently use low blood sugars as an opportunity to binge-eat everything in sight, it's time to acknowledge that self-destructive habit.

Yes, there are moments when we're simply trying to anticipate and guess and we guess wrong. It happens. But the habit of eating hundreds or thousands of calories multiple times a week during low blood sugars is a habit that is inevitably preventing you from thriving.

You do have control over how much you eat during a low blood sugar. Yes, your brain is begging you to eat more and more and more, but you *know* in your very brilliant mind that you do not need 250 grams of carbohydrates (and 1,000+ calories) to treat the average low blood sugar.

This habit of over-eating during lows leads to blood sugar roller coasters, guilt, shame, frustration, and weight gain. You have the power to change this habit — and you'll be glad you did!

A few tips to start changing this habit:

- **Stop using foods you really love to treat lows.** Instead, choose foods that you'll label as "medicine" to treat lows — like the fast-acting carbohydrates listed below. And then save the brownies or the ice cream for a moment of the day when you can truly enjoy it, take insulin for it, and eat it thoughtfully. (This of course, also means you'll want to consider nixing any intensely restrictive diets that have taught you to think of brownies or ice cream as "bad foods" instead of simply treats.) Remember, dietary fat and protein slow down the digestion of carbohydrates, so using high-fat foods means you're going to be low and feel lousy longer.

- **Treat the low, then distract your brain.** Drink a glass of water, chew some gum, nosh some carrots, or listen to three of your favorite songs while sitting on your hands. It's all about letting the carbs you ate actually digest, letting those symptoms calm down, and giving your body time to recover before you mindlessly consume 1,000 calories when you only needed 75 calories. Give yourself 15 minutes to start feeling better before you decide to eat more food.

- **Remind yourself: "I am in control of how much food I eat during this low."** Stop telling yourself that you're helpless, that you can't control it. You can. Take a deep breath and be rational. You're in charge. You're powerful! You're awesome! You're brilliant. You have the power to say, "Suzie, you've treated the low, now chill out and let those carbs do their job." Sure, there might be a rare low blood sugar here or there that truly requires 60+ grams of carbs because of way too much IOB, but generally, it's just unlikely.

- **Sure, the occasional low in the middle of exercise might need more than 15 grams of carbohydrates.** If you're in the middle of a jog with too much IOB, then yes, you might need a bigger treatment for that low. But that still doesn't mean binge-eating everything in the cupboard when you get home. Take a deep breath and treat your lows using your logic rather than fear and impulse. You'll thank yourself in the hours that follow.

- **If you do over-treat the low, forgive yourself immediately!** Yes, the urge to "rage bolus" after eating an entire pint of ice cream is pretty intense, but this is your next opportunity to take charge. Calculate your "rage bolus" and then *don't take it — because* *it's probably way too much.* Instead, take a deep breath (yes, another one) and *immediately* forgive yourself for over-eating. Your next goal is to be *safe.* Calculate a *careful bolus* and then distract yourself for the next couple of hours as you allow that insulin to start working. No, it won't be smooth and easy — considering you just consumed 200 grams of carbohydrates in one sitting — but it will feel a lot better than a wild roller coaster of extreme lows followed by extreme highs.

You are in charge of how much food you consume during a mild-to-moderate low blood sugar. Embrace that fact and free yourself from the self-destructive (and exhausting) habits of over-eating during lows.

Overtreating lows is such a common habit. We've all done it. But with a little persistence and patience, you can totally evolve this part of your diabetes management.

Be prepared for lows — always

Whether you're at the gym, on an easy 1-mile dog walk, or you're kayaking along your favorite river, you *must* carry at least 30 to 60 grams of carbohydrates with you. And if possible, emergency glucagon.

That may sound like a lot but some lows only require 8 grams of carbohydrates and others might require 45 grams. It depends on how much insulin is on board during that low, what kind of exercise you're doing, and how far you are from home.

Choose fast-acting carbohydrates that are easy to carry, don't melt, and don't freeze. Fast-acting means it breaks down quickly — which means it shouldn't contain fat or protein.

- Glucose tabs
- Glucose gel
- Energy gels
- Smarties (in the USA)
- Fruit juice
- Honey packets

- Maple syrup packets
- Jelly beans
- Skittles
- Sour Patch Kids
- Pixi Stix
- Airheads

This list could go on and on. Just keep in mind that the smaller the candy is, the more easily you can carry enough to treat more than one low or enough to treat a severe low.

Be prepared for *severe* lows, too

Exercise — and the hours that follow — creates a great opportunity for severe low blood sugar. Defined as blood sugar levels below 55 mg/dL or a low you cannot treat with food or beverage for any reason, severe low blood sugars are the scariest of the scary.

That's why we should *all* own emergency glucagon if possible. (There are a variety of discount coupons and copay cards for every brand of emergency glucagon available! Talk to your pharmacist!)

Even if you've *never* needed emergency glucagon, I urge you to ask your doctor for a prescription and fill it. Some of today's modern 1-step glucagon options even allow you to "micro-dose" glucagon which means you can take a small amount.

Emergency glucagon is intended to be used on you by someone else when you're unconscious, unresponsive, or seizing. (And you should definitely teach family and friends when and how to use emergency glucaon!)

First: if you or a loved one isn't sure of what to do, *call 911.*

However, you might use emergency glucagon on yourself if:

- You have a stomach virus and can't keep food down
- You accidentally took the wrong type of insulin
- You accidentally took the wrong dose of insulin

- Your blood sugar is plummeting in the middle of a 6-mile jog and you're terrified

- Your blood sugar is plummeting after dosing for a post-workout meal and you're terrified

- You believe you're going to lose consciousness — then call 911!

Today's modern 1-step emergency glucagon options include:

- **Gvoke HypoPen**: an auto-injector pen you press against your thigh

- **Gvoke Prefilled Syringe (PFS)**: a prefilled syringe you manually inject into your thigh

- **Zegalogue Glucagon Pen**: an auto-injector pen you press against your thigh

- **Baqsimi Nasal Glucagon:** a spray device that administers into your nose

The only option on this list that allows micro-dosing during exercise is the Gvoke Prefilled Syringe. The other options administer a full dose of glucagon. The Gvoke PFS prescription also usually provides you with *several* syringes in one prescription which means you can store it in a variety of places.

Glucagon can come with some side effects that linger for a day or several. Nasal glucagon can cause intense vomiting immediately after dosing, and a few days of severe headaches. All glucagon can lead to very stubborn highs for a day or several because it triggers your liver to release stored sugar. That trigger doesn't exactly turn off just because you've recovered from the severe low.

Keep it in your gym bag, your fanny pack, your nightstand, your coat pocket, and your desk at work. Remember to consider the *temperature* of where you're storing it and to replace it with a new prescription each year when it expires. Then tell your family, friends, and coworkers where it's located, when you might need it, and how to use it!

Treating lows during exercise

Treating lows during exercise can be tricky because there are so many variables to consider.

- What's causing the low — how much extra insulin is causing the low?

- Do you need 5 grams, 15 grams, or 50 grams based on the cause of the low?

- How many carbs do you need if you plan to finish your workout?

- Or is your blood sugar dropping so rapidly that you truly need to stop, eat more, and rest?

What we know for sure, though, is this:

- You should absolutely be prepared *always* with fast-acting carbs while exercising

- You should *not* use this as an opportunity to go nuts and eat *all the carbs*

- You should consider calling 911 or using emergency glucagon if the low is more than you can manage safely with food, if you're struggling to stay on your feet, if you're feeling like you might pass out

- You should *stop* exercise when you're low and treat the low thoughtfully

- You should choose fat-free/fast-acting carbs to treat lows while exercising

- You should give yourself at least 10-15 minutes for your blood sugar to rise before restarting

- You should consider how much insulin is still active in your system before restarting

- If you intend to eventually continue exercising, you might find it helpful to eat a more substantial carb-source after the fast-acting carbs — like a small yogurt or a granola bar — to slowly soak up the extra IOB.

The more consistent and thoughtful you are in how you manage lows during exercise, the more likely you'll recover smoothly without a dramatic rebound — and eventually continue exercising!

Don't panic. Be thoughtful. Call 911 or treat with emergency glucagon if needed.

Lows can be scary. But we are powerful!

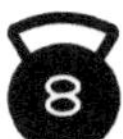

Weight-loss tips with type 1 diabetes

Losing or maintaining your weight with T1D is not easy. And there's a good reason for it.

You already know your body doesn't produce insulin properly — but you might not know that your body *also* doesn't produce *five* other hormones properly!

When your T1D immune system mistakenly attacks the pancreas, it's attacking the islet cells. Islet cells are responsible for the production of:

- Insulin
- Amylin
- Ghrelin
- Glucagon
- Pancreatic polypeptide
- Somatostatin

These hormones are pretty darn important when it comes to managing your weight! These hormones regulate a variety of things, including:

- Your blood sugar after eating by slowing down the process of digestion
- Suppressing liver glucose production — which then reduces insulin needs
- Signaling to your brain that you are full during/after eating
- Managing your hour-by-hour appetite
- Extra glucose from your liver means extra insulin which means

> extra glucose to store as body fat

- ...and more!

These all play a huge role in your body's ability to maintain its weight! Your brain isn't getting cues that your stomach is full? Holy moly! That seems pretty critical!

Your stomach is digesting food more quickly than the human body is supposed to? That might explain why it's so darn hard to prevent big spikes after eating! (And why we probably need more insulin to manage a meal than a non-diabetic body!)

Your liver is producing more glucose *all the time* than it needs to? And then insulin takes the excess glucose and stores it as body fat? Well, *geez*, this all seems like a recipe for weight gain, rising insulin needs, and an insatiable appetite.

And there are medications to address those other hormones — more on *that* in a moment. Here are a few tips to help you lose or maintain your weight as a person living with T1D.

Get real about what you're eating

Listen, I eat dessert on a daily basis. And as much as I'd like to say, "Sure, we can eat anything!", it's important to acknowledge that we cannot get away with as much as the non-diabetic eater.

I'm not suggesting your diet needs to be perfect — and I'm definitely not suggesting that you need to start an extremely restrictive diet. I'm simply suggesting the idea that we need to hold ourselves even more accountable than those who produce plenty of insulin and amylin.

If you're eating pizza and fast food on a regular frequency of any kind, you're going to struggle with your weight. If you're stopping at a fast-food breakfast joint every morning for scones and *coffee-drinks-that-are-actually-dessert*, you're going to struggle with your weight. If you're rarely cooking fresh food for yourself — which means you're eating a lot of processed/pre-packaged products — you're going to struggle with your weight.

If you want to face your weight-loss goals, you've got to face how much low-quality food you're consuming.

It doesn't even have to require tons of cooking! For your daytime meals, grab more whole foods, for example: fruit + veggie + fat = apple + carrots + hummus + nuts. Keep it simple. Save your cooking energy/time for the evening.

Adopting a 90/10 or 80/20 approach to nutrition will make a big difference. The 90 or the 80 implies the food that you're mostly eating throughout the day — and in this case, I'm suggesting you make 90 or 80 percent of what you eat very, very healthy wholesome choices.

The 10 or 20 percent is the treats that prevent feelings of deprivation and vengeful binge-eating. Whether it's pizza or cupcakes or potato chips, you're creating *room* in your diet for those less-than-perfect foods that you just love and crave and enjoy. You're not cutting them entirely from your diet. You're simply making room for them by ensuring that *most of* what you eat is really high-quality, real food.

Check out intermittent fasting

Intermittent fasting is the practice of intentionally *not* eating for certain hours of the day and consuming your day's worth of calories in other specific hours of the day.

Yes, it's a trendy thing, but intermittent fasting (IF) can be really helpful for people with T1D — and I know many T1Ds who've adopted it as a major part of their lifelong lifestyle. I started practicing IF a few months after my first child was born — to deal with a stubborn eight pounds that wouldn't budge.

Here are two places to find great guidance on IF:

- Precisionnutrition.com/intermittent-fasting by Dr. John Berardi
- Diabetesstrong.com/intermittent-fasting-type-1-diabetes by Ginger Vieira

We've already talked *so much* about fasting in this book that IF will be relatively easy to grasp. In a nutshell, you skip breakfast and don't eat your first meal until at least 12 or 1 p.m. If your basal/background insulin doses are properly fine-tuned, you'll likely find that your blood sugar *rises* and you need a fairly scheduled dose of rapid-acting insulin between waking up and eating lunch.

For me, I need a ½ unit of rapid-acting injected insulin around 8 a.m to account for dawn phenomenon hormones that trigger my liver to release stored glucose. In the past, I've needed another around 11 a.m. (Taking a GLP-1 medication as described later in this chapter can help suppress that liver glucose.)

There are five reasons IF is so helpful for people with T1D:

1. **It immediately eliminates several hundred calories from your day.** You should make sure you're still eating *enough* but the reduction of even just 400 calories per day can easily lead to a 2 to 3-pound weight loss per month! Stick with it and you're well on your way to achieving patient, sustainable weight loss.

2. **It hugely reduces the amount of time you spend in the day thinking about food and blood sugar levels.** You literally don't have to worry about breakfast screwing up your day because you *didn't* eat breakfast. Sure, you might need a small bolus to deal with the glucose your liver produces because you skipped breakfast, but that's way easier than managing whatever you might have purchased at a fast-food chain on your way to work.

3. **It reduces your appetite.** Okay, don't be surprised if you *freak out* during the first week and overeat when your fasting window ends. Take a deep breath — it's okay. If you can give yourself room to experiment, you might eventually find that the panic of "Oh my goodness, I'm so hungry!" dissipates and you just enjoy the lightness of being in that fasted state. You might find that you're not starving to death. That is okay. And you feel good when do finally "break the fast" at 1 p.m. with a very wholesome meal made with *real* food instead of pizza.

4. **Exercising during this fasted state can be *a lot* easier than trying to time your workout after a normal meal with a bolus of insulin.** So many people with T1D already engage in different types of workouts along with IF for this very reason. It's a funny feeling at first — exercising without having eaten — but if you get past the "I'm gonna starve!" panic, you may find you really en-

joy it. Of course, be prepared for lows, take notes, adjust, and try again as needed. If you go low, you should *definitely* break the fast and treat your low thoughtfully. If you don't *over-treat* the low, you can continue fasting at least in terms of not taking a bolus of insulin. Perfect? No. But it's not a big deal. Treat the low and move on!

5. **In general, IF can calm down this constant worry about lows and food.** It's just a break from the non-stop battle of insulin vs. food. It goes against everything we've been taught — but it can be really life-changing. So many of the people I know who've tried it have adopted it as a core lifestyle for *most* days of the week because it simply feels good and makes part of the day with T1D a bit easier. If you don't stick to it seven days a week, *it's okay.*

Here are a few common IF schedules:

Schedule type	Fasting window	Eating window	Example
16:8	16 hours	8 hours	Fasting 10pm to 1pm
14:10	14 hours	10 hours	Fasting 10pm to 11am
24 hours once per week	24 hours (1 day)	6 days per usual	Fasting on Sunday Breakfast on Monday

I recommend a 16:8 or 14:10 schedule — especially for newbies.

Regardless, don't go crazy over it. This isn't a cult. Listen to your body and create an approach to IF that you can maintain.

For example, if you find IF works well Monday through Friday but you want to have pancakes with your kids or brunch with your pals on the weekend, *then fine — eat breakfast.* If you cave in on a Tuesday and eat at 10 a.m. instead of 1 p.m., it's *okay.* If you practice IF for six months and suddenly find yourself truly needing to eat breakfast every day, *then fine — eat breakfast.*

You might learn that you need a reduced basal setting during fasting or you might learn you need a bit more basal during fasting. It really depends on your current basal settings (if they are as minimal as possible) and how much glucose your liver releases in response to skipping breakfast. Take notes! Be thoughtful. Check your blood sugar often.

You don't have to be a hardcore nut to gain benefits from IF. Step away from these dogmatic insane rules that it's all or nothing. Listen to your body. Experiment. Choose mostly real food. Try new things. Check your blood sugar. If you need to treat a low or correct a high, do it thoughtfully and move on. It's okay.

Consider a GLP-1 medication

It's not cheating. Instead, it's giving your body medication to compensate *for the other hormones* you're not producing.

GLP-1 medications include brand names like Ozempic (semaglutide) and Trulicity (dulaglutide). These drugs help do the things that those other five hormones would do for you! While they're currently FDA-approved for use in people with type 2 diabetes, there are *so many* people with T1D taking these medications that it's being studied intensely for their use in T1D, too.

- GLP-1 medications slow down how quickly your meal empties into your bloodstream — reducing that post-meal blood sugar spike.

- GLP-1 medications increase your body's sensitivity to insulin — which helps you need less insulin to achieve the same blood sugar level goals. This inevitably means less glucose is being stored as fat.

- GLP-1 medications reduce the amount of glucose your liver produces — which inevitably means you're storing less glucose as body fat and reduces your insulin needs.

- GLP-1 medications help you feel full sooner after eating — which helps you eat less and feel more satisfied after eating.

- **Read more**: T1Dexchange.org/semaglutide-type-1-diabetes

While there have been medications intentionally designed to replace amylin (brand name, Symlin), they weren't very successful because they required multiple daily injections, the impact on blood sugar wasn't particularly steady or predictable, and the side effects were a bit severe — including intense nausea and vomiting.

GLP-1 medications have proven to be more easily tolerated and gentler on your stomach. (The side effects often dissipate within the first couple of weeks.) GLP-1 medications usually require a once-weekly injection, making them easy to add to your diabetes management routine. There is an oral version, too, named Rybelsus.

There's no shame in taking insulin, right? There shouldn't be shame associated with taking medication to compensate for the other hormones you're not producing properly.

These medications *can be* expensive out-of-pocket, though. Getting it covered by private insurance shouldn't be too difficult if your endocrinologist is explaining that you're struggling with weight loss, insulin resistance, and post-meal blood sugar spikes.

Get moving — every day

Make it a priority. Your body needs exercise — every day. Some days you might only have time for a 30-minute powerwalk instead of a trip to the gym, and that's okay! In fact, that's *great*.

There's really no reason we shouldn't be exercising nearly every single day as people with T1D. Your body needs all the help it can get to maintain insulin sensitivity. Daily exercise will play a huge role in helping you thrive with this disease.

Exercise has proven to increase energy, self-esteem, and joy! Why wouldn't you want to get in on *that*?

Make it happen. Make it a priority. Make it your religion! If other busy people with jobs and kids have figured out how to fit it in, you can, too! No more excuses. You can make this a real part of your life if you choose to do so. (P.s. I watch trashy reality dating shows while I jump rope in the morning! Please don't tell anybody! It's so entertaining.)

Let's talk about the booze and wine...

Oh, I love a delicious glass of wine or one of those fruit vodka seltzer things — but if you're drinking alcohol most nights of the week as a person with T1D, you're going to struggle with your weight.

It's about balance. It's about setting parameters. Alcohol is poison. Seriously — when you consume any type of alcohol, your liver stops breaking down food and absorbing vitamins and just says, "Whoa! Poison is present! I must deal with this until it's out!"

It's a treat. It's something we should set boundaries around for a huge number of reasons, and weight management is just *one* of those reasons.

Are you using alcohol to "wind down" after a usual day at work — every day?

It's time to get real about your alcohol consumption. Alcohol promotes belly fat. Alcohol contributes to depression. Alcohol contributes to feeling lethargic the next morning. Alcohol contributes to over-eating. Alcohol might be keeping you from feeling *well enough* to exercise the next day. Alcohol can be a crutch instead of a treat.

Track your diet/exercise for a little while — but don't get obsessed

Whether you're tracking exercise or carbohydrates or alcohol, tracking can be so helpful for getting a new habit established. But just because you track your calorie intake for three weeks doesn't mean you need to do it *forever*.

Use that process to learn more about your current habits and help you shape new ones. It's really, really okay if you don't want to track every darn calorie for the rest of eternity.

Personally, I like tracking my exercise on a big marker board every week because it helps me feel productive! I love writing it down. The process is *always* rewarding for me — which tells me it's a positive tracking process rather than a demotivating or stressful one.

Experiment. Learn. Move on when it's time!

Stop dieting — seriously

Just stop. Stop trying to omit entire categories of macronutrients (carbs or fat, for example) from your diet. Stop re-starting the same strict diet over and over that clearly isn't working for you if you have to keep re-starting it. Stop expecting an extreme diet to result in rapid weight loss, then return to your previous habits, and discover the weight returns instantly.

Just stop with the crazy yo-yo dieting. Instead, take a good hard look at your core habits around nutrition and exercise. Then vow to start *experimenting* with small adjustments — like eating more real food, making indulgent choices like fast food a rare treat, and listening more closely to how your body *feels* based on what you just ate.

Stop trying to force somebody else's crazy diet down your own throat. You can learn so much from *experimenting*. You might learn how to eat fewer processed carbs or eat more vegetables. You might learn that you're overeating at lunch or stress eating at night.

You probably already know that strict ketogenic diets don't work for you — but that doesn't mean you can't learn how to eat *fewer* processed carbs. It doesn't have to be all or nothing. It doesn't have to be extreme.

Experiment without judgment. Learn from it. Move on.

Like Bruce Lee said, "Take what is useful and leave the rest."

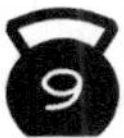

The cool down chapter

It's a lot of work — exercising with T1D. Actually, it's a lot of work to just get through another day with this disease.

Hand this book to that relative who keeps saying, "Oh, that little pager in your pocket does everything for you, right?" and their brain might explode. (Well, after they offer you some sugar-free chocolates and remind you about their diabetic cat. RIP ol' Mr. Whiskers.)

You are a T1D powerhouse. Resilient as heck. The intensity of what you have to do simply to survive a brief walk with your dog proves it. You're a survivor. A warrior. An hour-by-hour champion of a life-threatening game. It probably sounds quite dramatic to many, but it's the truth: every hour that you've kept yourself alive is another hour you've won.

You've gotten so used to this non-stop reality that you don't even realize how impressive it is.

Perhaps I'm in a particularly feisty mood this morning as I type this — but if I'm being honest, I like people with T1D more than I like anybody else. There's a good reason why people with T1D bond so quickly and intensely with each other. People with this disease know: despite how cute celebrities with T1D make it look in commercials, it is brutal work to learn, manage, and endure.

And that's if you're lucky enough to have enough insulin, can afford the latest CGM or insulin pump, and have access to a knowledgeable and supportive healthcare team.

We could devote an entire book to the exhausting burden of trying to *pay* for the things you need in order to actually stay alive with T1D.

Now get ready for my Tony Robbins/Oprah Winfrey pep talk, because it's coming. Okay, here it is:

If you're fortunate to have the critical basics (insulin, tech, health care), then you have two choices in this obnoxious disease:

- **Option 1:** Get mad. Live in a state of constant frustration. Blame yourself. Blame the world. Give up. Do the bare minimum to keep yourself alive and wrap yourself up in a big cozy bubble of anger for years to come.

- **Option 2:** Get mad. Take a deep breath. Take another deep breath. Take notes. Learn a little bit more. Try again.

And remember, if your usual T1D exercise plan suddenly starts causing lows, it *doesn't* mean exercise is evil! It probably just means one of the other dozens of variables that affect your insulin needs has changed — and you need to make some adjustments.

Type 1 diabetes is not fun. Ever — well, except for when you meet cool people who also have T1D and you instantly admire each other because you know they *know* how hard you work to stay alive. If I could get my hands on the latest stem-cell therapy currently in human trials, I'd be like, "Hook me up! Let's see what happens!"

Surely, you get my point: this isn't easy. We wake up and we do what we have to in order to live. This book, I hope, inspires you to wake up and do what you can to *thrive*.

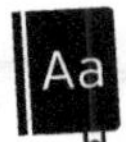

Words & phrases you need to know

Here are a few words or phrases you need to know before reading this book. These words or phrases will be explained in greater detail within the context of the book — some even have their own dedicated chapters!

Aerobic exercise

Cardio exercise is a type of physical activity performed at an intensity you can sustain without stopping for an extended period of time.

Anaerobic exercise

Commonly known as high-intensity exercises or strength training, a type of physical activity performed at an intensity that can only be performed in short bursts.

Bolus insulin

A dose of rapid-acting insulin taken to cover meals or to correct high blood sugar.

Basal/background insulin

Insulin that covers your background insulin needs delivered via an insulin pump (with basal rates) or an injection of long-acting insulin.

Carbohydrates

Carbohydrates are one of the three macronutrients carbohydrates, fat, and protein in the food you eat. While all three can affect blood sugar levels and insulin needs, carbohydrates usually have the most dramatic impact on blood sugar levels and require the most planning for insulin dosing and blood sugar management.

Closed-loop insulin pump

Also referred to as "looping", closed-loop pumps are insulin pumps that communicate directly with your continuous glucose monitor (CGM) and automatically make adjustments in your insulin dosages in an effort to prevent fluctuations. Brand names include Omnipod 5, Tandem t:Slim, and Medtronic 670G and 770G.

Continuous glucose monitor (CGM)

Diabetes technology that measures blood sugar levels without pricking your finger. Brand names include Freestyle Libre, Dexcom, and Eversense. CGMs are highly recommended for anyone living with type 1 diabetes.

Correction dose

The insulin you take to correct high blood sugar levels.

Diabetic ketoacidosis (DKA) / ketones

This is a life-threatening condition caused by too little insulin and usually accompanied by very high blood sugars. While there are safe circumstances in which ketones are present (nutritional ketosis, for example), ketones caused by too little insulin in your body can lead to severe vomiting, dehydration, coma, and death. Talk to your healthcare team to get ketone strips for measuring ketone levels during high blood sugars, illness, etc.

Fasted exercise

Exercising when you don't have a dose of insulin in your system for a meal.

Glucose

The sugar in your blood stream! In this book, we use "blood sugar" or "blood glucose" to both imply the level on your CGM or your glucose meter.

Glucagon

A hormone produced by the pancreas that tells your liver to release stored glucose. In those without T1D, your body naturally produces glucagon between meals and to prevent low blood sugar during exercise. In those of us with T1D, this natural regulation of glucagon is dysfunctional. Emergency glucagon kits contain a large dose of glucose to be administered during severe hypoglycemia. A large dose of glucagon tells your liver to release a large amount of stored glucose to bring your blood sugar back up to a safe level.

Goal range/target range

Your personal blood sugar goals. The standard recommended target range by the American Diabetes Association is 80 to 180 mg/dL. The more you learn about blood sugar management, the tighter your target range might become. You may have a looser target range due to fear of hypoglycemia, inability to feel symptoms of hypoglycemia, your age, etc. That's okay! Your goal range should be thoughtfully decided with support from your healthcare team to help you be as safe and healthy as you can.

Hypoglycemia / Low blood sugar

Blood sugar levels below 70 mg/dL. Throughout this book, I will refer to hypoglycemia as low blood sugar. Severe low blood sugar is generally considered anything below 55 mg/dL when your risk of losing consciousness or experiencing a seizure increases significantly.

Hyperglycemia / high blood sugar

Also known as hyperglycemia, blood sugar levels above your goal range. For some, that's over 150 mg/dL, and for others, it's over 225 mg/dL Throughout this book, I will refer to hyperglycemia as high blood sugar, with a level of 180 mg/dL as the general standard. What qualifies as high blood sugar can vary greatly from person-to-person depending on your personal comfort levels, access to newer diabetes technology and medications, and goals. Exercising with blood sugar levels over 250 mg/dL can increase your risk of developing ketones — talk to your healthcare team about reasonable goals for you!

Insulin-on-board (IOB)

The insulin that is already active in your body. Mostly, IOB talks about rapid-acting insulin delivered via injection, pump, or inhalation. IOB includes both bolus and basal insulin.

Inhaled insulin

One of the newer insulins on the market that delivers ultra-rapid-acting insulin via oral inhalation. For simplicity throughout this book, I will include inhaled insulin as part of rapid-acting insulin discussions. Brand names include Afrezza. Read more at GingerVieira.com/diabetes.

Insulin sensitivity/insulin resistance

Your body's need for insulin can vary based on increasing insulin resistance (which means you need more insulin to manage in-range blood sugar levels) or increasing insulin sensitivity (which means you need less insulin to manage in-range blood sugar levels. Neither one is completely good or completely bad. There are many natural factors that can cause a body to become more insulin resistant — like growth hormones, reproductive hormones, excitement, stress, etc. Other factors are typically less desirable — like weight gain, lack of physical activity, a diet high in processed fatty foods, excessive stress, smoking cigarettes, drinking too much caffeine, and too little sleep. Increasing your insulin sensitivity is usually ideal because the less insulin you need to manage in-range blood sugar levels, the easier it will likely be. Factors that can increase insulin sensitivity include losing weight, regular exercise, a cleaner diet, adequate sleep, limited caffeine, and manageable stress levels.

Intermittent fasting

An approach to eating during certain times of day and not eating during others. The most popular is a 16:8 approach which means you fast for 16 hours and eat your day's worth of calories within 8 hours. Many people approach this by eating their last meal before bed and not eating again until the next afternoon around 1 or 2 p.m.

Long-acting insulin

Insulin that is taken once or twice a day to serve your basal/background insulin needs. Every person with type 1 diabetes needs basal/background insulin of some kind at all times. Brand names include Lantus, Toujeo, Tresiba, Lyumjev, and Levemir.

Pancreas

The organ responsible for producing insulin, amylin, glucagon, and much more! This is the organ that your immune system is attacking as a person with T1D. Technically, your pancreas is healthy but your immune system is dysfunctional.

Rapid-acting insulin

Insulin that begins working within an hour and stays in your system for anywhere from 3 to 6 hours. It can be used via a pump for both basal and bolus insulin doses. Can be used via pen or syringe for bolus insulin needs. Brand names include Novolog, Humalog, Fiasp, Apidra, Admelog, and Afrezza (inhaled, ultra-rapid).

Type 1 diabetes

A chronic illness defined by an autoimmune attack on the cells of your pancreas that produce insulin and several other critical hormones. T1D also includes latent autoimmune deficiency in adults (LADA) and can develop at any age. There are actually six hormones people with T1D don't produce properly — more on this in Chapter 7! There is no cure at this time. Recent FDA approval of the drug teplizumab has shown to delay the full onset of T1D if its administered in the earliest stages of the disease.

Type 2 diabetes

A metabolic disorder defined by insulin resistance and dysfunctional insulin production. People with T2D may struggle to produce normal amounts of insulin or properly use the insulin they do produce. Contrary to mainstream media, it is not caused by sugary diets or weight gain but lifestyle habits can play a role in the development of the disease. A significant percentage of people with T2D cannot simply reverse the condition through diet and weightloss.

Keep Learning

Thriving with T1D is all about learning. Here are a handful of resources from awesome experts in the diabetes community to continue your T1D education:

- The Athlete's Guide to Diabetes by Sheri Colberg, PhD
- Think Like a Pancreas by Gary Scheiner, MS, CDCES
- Sugar Surfing by Stephen Ponder, MD, FAACP, CDCES
- Bright Spots and Landmines by Adam Brown
- Dealing with Diabetes Burnout by Ginger Vieira
- Emotional Eating with Diabetes by Ginger Vieira
- Fit with Diabetes (ebook) by Christel Oerum
- Risely Health (coaching): RiselyHealth.com
- Your Diabetes Insider (coaching): YourDiabetesInsider.com
- Integrated Diabetes Services (coaching): IntegratedDiabetes.com

NEVER

GIVE UP!

YOU'VE GOT THIS.

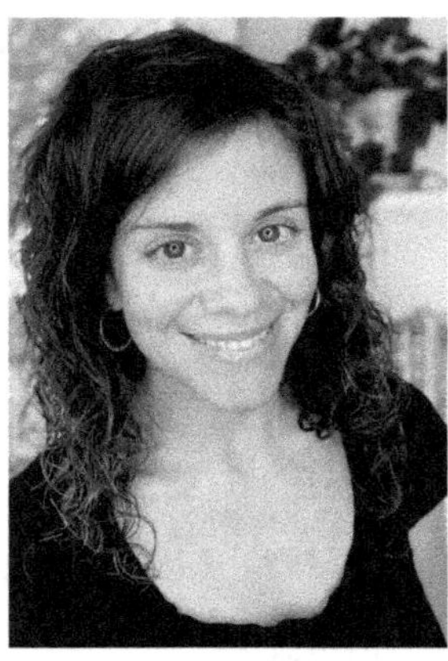

About the author

Ginger Vieira has lived with type 1 diabetes and celiac disease since 1999 and fibromyalgia since 2014. She is the author of several books available on Amazon, including:

- Pregnancy with Type 1 Diabetes
- Dealing with Diabetes Burnout
- Emotional Eating with Diabetes
- When I Go Low (for kids)
- Ain't Gonna Hide My T1D! (for kids)

Ginger Vieira has lived with type 1 diabetes since 1999. She also lives with celiac disease, fibromyalgia, hypothyroidism, and POTS. She is thriving and loving life! Once upon a time, Ginger was a personal trainer, yoga instructor, and competitive powerlifter. Today, Ginger creates educational diabetes articles and videos for a variety of companies. She lives with two beautiful kiddos, a handsome fella, and two dogs in Vermont.

Find more from Ginger at GingerVieira.com and YouTube.com/@ DiabetesNerd.

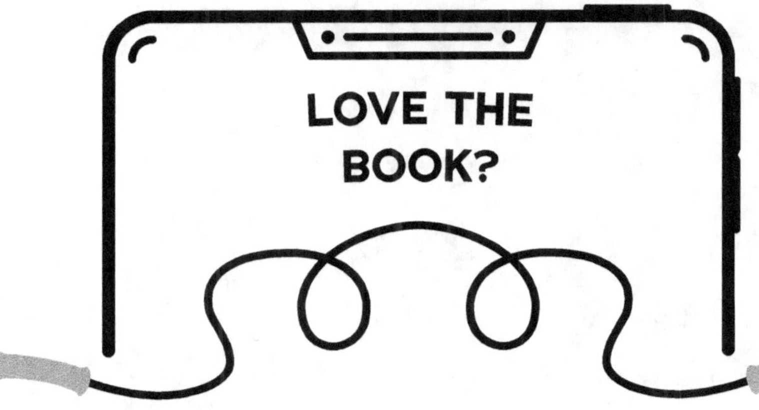

LEAVE A REVIEW ON AMAZON!

This book was self-published.

**Reviews and social media posts
make a big difference!**